Ocular Photodynamic Therapy

Ocular Photodynamic Therapy

Carmen A. Puliafito, MD, MBA
Bascom Palmer Eye Institute
University of Miami School of Medicine
Miami, Florida

Adam H. Rogers, MD
New England Eye Center
Tufts University School of Medicine
Boston, Massachusetts

Adam Martidis, MD
Wills Eye Hospital
Jefferson Medical College
Philadelphia, Pennsylvania

Paul B. Greenberg, MD
Bascom Palmer Eye Institute
University of Miami School of Medicine
Miami, Florida

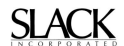

SLACK
INCORPORATED

an innovative information, education, and management company
6900 Grove Road • Thorofare, NJ 08086

The procedures and practices described in this book should be implemented in a manner consistent with the professional standards set for the circumstances that apply in each specific situation. Every effort has been made to confirm the accuracy of the information presented and to correctly relate generally accepted practices. The author, editor, and publisher cannot accept responsibility for errors or exclusions or for the outcome of the application of the material presented herein. There is no expressed or implied warranty of this book or information imparted by it.

Care has been taken to ensure that drug selection and dosages are in accordance with currently accepted/recommended practice. Due to continuing research, changes in government policy and regulations, and various effects of drug reactions and interactions, it is recommended that the reader review all materials and literature provided for each drug, especially those that are new or not frequently used.

Any review or mention of specific companies or products is not intended as an endorsement by the author or the publisher.

Ocular photodynamic therapy / Carmen A. Puliafito ... [et al.].
      p. ; cm.
    ISBN 1-55642-490-6 (alk. paper)
    1. Retinal degeneration--Photochemotherapy. 2. Choroid--Diseases--Photochemotherapy. 3. Neovascularization. I. Puliafito, Carmen A.
    [DNLM: 1. Choroidal Neovascularization--therapy. 2. Macular Degeneration--therapy. 3. Photography--methods. WW 245 O21 2002]
    RE661 .M3 O28 2002
    617.7'35--dc21

                                                                    2001042942

Printed in the United States of America

Published by: SLACK Incorporated
                     6900 Grove Road
                     Thorofare, NJ 08086 USA
                     Telephone: 856-848-1000
                     Fax: 856-853-5991
                     www.slackbooks.com

    Contact SLACK Incorporated for more information about other books in this field or about the availability of our books from distributors outside the United States.
    Authorization to photocopy items for internal or personal use, or the internal or personal use of specific clients, is granted by SLACK Incorporated, provided that the appropriate fee is paid directly to Copyright Clearance Center, 222 Rosewood Drive, Danvers, MA 01923 USA, 978-750-8400. Prior to photocopying items for educational classroom use, please contact the CCC at the address above. Please reference Account Number 9106324 for SLACK Incorporated's Professional Book Division.
    For further information on CCC, check CCC Online at the following address: http://www.copyright.com.

    Last digit is print number: 10 9 8 7 6 5 4 3 2 1

DEDICATION

This book is dedicated to the staff, photographers, and patients of the New England Eye Center, who made this book possible.

CONTENTS

About the Authors

Carmen A. Puliafito, MD, MBA
Glaser Professor and Chair, Department of Ophthalmology
Bascom Palmer Eye Institute
University of Miami School of Medicine
Miami, Fla

Medical Director
Anne Bates Leach Eye Hospital
Miami, Fla

Former Director
New England Eye Center
Professor and Chair, Department of Ophthalmology
Tufts University School of Medicine
Boston, Mass

Adam H. Rogers, MD
Assistant Professor of Ophthalmology
New England Eye Center
Tufts University School of Medicine
Boston, Mass

Adam Martidis, MD
Instructor of Ophthalmology
Wills Eye Hospital
Jefferson Medical College
Philadelphia, Pa

Paul B. Greenberg, MD
Assistant Professor of Clinical Ophthalmology
Bascom Palmer Eye Institute
University of Miami School of Medicine
Miami, Fla

PREFACE

Photodynamic therapy (PDT) of choroidal neovascularization (CNV) represents a major advancement in the treatment of age-related macular degeneration. While earlier therapies focused on ablation of CNV with destruction of the surrounding neurosensory retina, PDT works in a more selective fashion, minimizing collateral damage to the retina.

Ocular Photodynamic Therapy represents our cumulative clinical experience with this treatment modality at the New England Eye Center. The focus of this book is to introduce photodynamic therapy to all ophthalmologists. For clinicians interested in learning about using PDT, a review of practical treatment conventions is provided. Experienced clinicians will benefit from the authors' insights into finer points of patient management, such as retreatment decisions or the role of optical coherence tomography. Practical examples underscore the indications, limitations, and potential complications of PDT. Expanded indications for lesions that do not meet strict study criteria are also reviewed.

PDT is not a cure for age-related macular degeneration, and new treatment modalities are on the horizon as this book is being published. The cases presented herein use verteporfin as the photosensitizing agent, as it is the only commercially available drug at present. New photosensitizing agents are currently in Phase II/III trials and have slightly different properties than verteporfin. How these drugs will differ from verteporfin will be determined with clinical trials and widespread use by clinicians.

Carmen A. Puliafito, MD, MBA
Adam H. Rogers, MD
Adam Martidis, MD
Paul B. Greenberg, MD

CHAPTER ONE

AGE-RELATED MACULAR DEGENERATION AND SUBFOVEAL CHOROIDAL NEOVASCULARIZATION

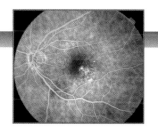 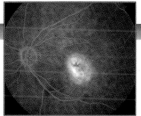 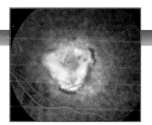

CHAPTER SECTIONS

- ❖ Classification of Age-Related Macular Degeneration
- ❖ Epidemiology
- ❖ Pathophysiology of Age-Related Macular Degeneration
- ❖ Natural History of Subfoveal Choroidal Neovascularization

Age-related macular degeneration (AMD) is the leading cause of central vision loss in individuals 65 years of age and older in developed countries.[1-4] The disease affects the choriocapillaris, Bruch's membrane, and retinal pigment epithelium (RPE) complex (Figure 1-1). Loss of vision ultimately occurs from photoreceptor damage due to the development of atrophic changes or choroidal neovascularization (CNV).[5] While most individuals are affected with the nonexudative type of AMD, patients with subfoveal CNV experience the most severe visual dysfunction. Given the impact of this disease and the expansion of the elderly population, extensive resources continue to be dedicated to the prevention and treatment of AMD.

CLASSIFICATION OF AGE-RELATED MACULAR DEGENERATION

AMD occurs in two forms: non-neovascular ("dry") and neovascular ("wet"). Non-neovascular AMD accounts for roughly 80% of all diagnosed cases.[3] In the Beaver Dam Eye Study among adults aged 43 to 86, non-neovascular AMD had a prevalence of 15.6% compared to 1.2% in neovascular AMD.[1] While the etiology is unknown, AMD occurs secondary to changes at the RPE-Bruch's membrane-choriocapillaris complex,[5,6] characterized by drusen, RPE degeneration, focal areas of hyperpigmentation, and geographic atrophy. Most patients presenting with drusen are visually asymptomatic. The presence of soft drusen in the fovea may cause decreased visual acuity and metamorphopsia (Figure 1-2). Geographic atrophy (Figure 1-3) is the most visually devastating manifestation of non-neovascular AMD and is responsible for up to 21% of reported cases of blindness secondary to AMD.[3]

Nearly 80% of all visual loss occurs from the formation of CNV.[3] This is a process involving the formation of abnormal choroidal blood vessels extending through defects in Bruch's membrane (Figure 1-4) to remain under the RPE layer (Type I CNV) or penetrating through the RPE into the retina (Type II CNV). CNV is classified into two major categories according to its appearance on fluorescein angiography: classic and occult CNV (Figures 1-5 and 1-6). These two forms of neovascular AMD may occur independent of one another, or neovascular lesions may angiographically exhibit characteristics of each.

On biomicroscopy, the appearance of classic CNV depends on the chronicity of the lesion. Classic CNV presenting in the acute stages clinically appears as a serous detachment of the neurosensory retina typically without subretinal hemorrhage or lipid exudation. Classic CNV that is more chronic clinically demonstrates subretinal fibrosis with varying degrees of subretinal hemorrhage and lipid exudation. A grayish-green subretinal elevation is often classically described. Classic CNV is angiographically defined as a well-demarcated area with early hyperfluorescence during the early phase of the angiogram with leakage of fluorescein during the venous and recirculation phases that obscures its border.[7]

Occult CNV clinically appears as a mottled elevation of the RPE. Subretinal fibrosis, subretinal hemorrhage, and lipid exudation may be present, but are usually identified in more chronic occult lesions. Occult CNV angiographically occurs in two patterns: fibrovascular pigment epithelial detachment (PED) and late leakage of undetermined origin.[8] Fibrovascular PED is described as stippled hyperfluorescence occurring at 1 to 2 minutes after fluorescein injection, with persistent late leakage. While the borders of an occult CNV primarily have poorly demarcated borders, a fibrovascular PED may have well-demarcated borders on fluorescein angiography. Late leakage of undetermined origin presents with areas of leakage occurring approximately between 2 and 5 minutes after the injection of fluorescein. The source of the fluorescein leakage is difficult to discern, and the boundaries of the lesion are always poorly demarcated.[8]

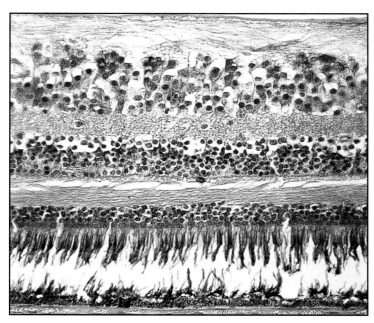

Figure 1-1. Histologic cross-section of a normal retina.

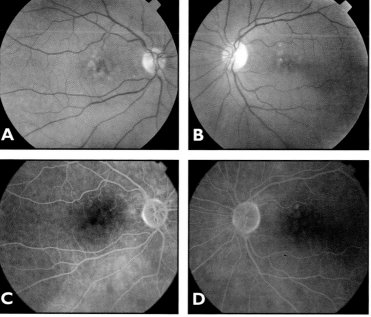

Figure 1-2. A 72-year-old female with soft drusen focused near the fovea and visual acuity measuring 20/50 OD and 20/30 OS. The patient complained of decreased vision attributed to foveal drusen (A and B). Fluorescein an-giography demonstrates staining of the drusen (C and D).

EPIDEMIOLOGY

Many epidemiological studies have evaluated the prevalence of AMD. Signs of macular degeneration may present as early as the fourth and fifth decades.[1,4,7,9] However, the onset of visual loss typically occurs between 65 and 75 years of age, with the incidence increasing with older age.[1,4,9,10] Determination of the actual prevalence of AMD is difficult to estimate as the definition varies among the studies (Table 1-1). Many studies combine geographic

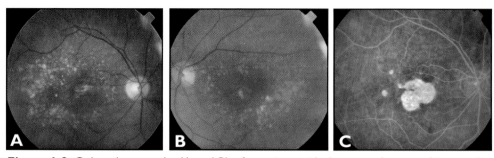

Figure 1-3. Color photographs (A and B) of a patient with drusen and geographic atrophy. Fluorescein angiography OD (C) demonstrates a window defect present in the area of geographic atrophy from the loss of the choriocapillaris and the RPE. Visual acuity measured 20/200 OD and 20/200 OS.

Figure 1-4. Histologic cross-section of CNV (courtesy of Nora Laver, MD).

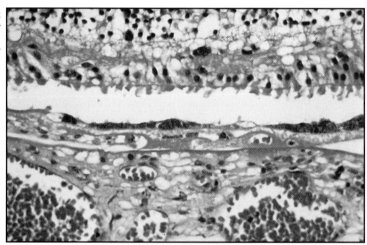

Figure 1-5. Classic CNV with well-delineated vessels and early hyperfluorescence (A). Late frames of the angiogram demonstrate diffuse leakage (B).

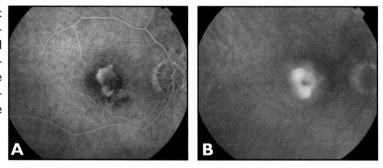

atrophy, a finding of dry AMD, and CNV into one group termed "late AMD." Other studies use the all-inclusive term AMD to lump dry and wet macular degeneration together.

The examining ophthalmologist and the expert reviewing the funduscopic photographs determined the diagnosis of AMD in a random sample of 3821 residents of Salisbury, Md, in the Salisbury Eye Evaluation Study. The prevalence of blindness (visual acuity 20/200 or worse) among white individuals with AMD was 0.38% in the 70- to 79-year-old age group, increasing to 1.15% in individuals aged 80 to 84 years.[2] The Baltimore Eye Survey evaluat-

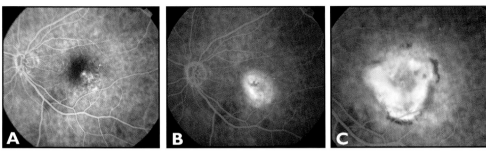

Figure 1-6. Occult CNV (A) was diagnosed when a 71-year-old female presented with metamorphopsia and decreased visual acuity of 20/60. Stippled hyperfluorescence was evident on the angiogram at baseline. At 1 month (B), the visual acuity declined to 20/80 with enlargement of the occult lesion. Five months after presentation (C), visual acuity was 20/250 with subretinal fibrosis and continued growth of the CNV.

TABLE 1-1				
PREVALENCE OF CHOROIDAL NEOVASCULARIZATION FROM AGE-RELATED MACULAR DEGENERATION IN POPULATION-BASED STUDIES				
Study	**Published (Year)**	**Participants (Number)**	**Age (Years)**	**Prevalence of Neovascular AMD (%)**
Beaver Dam Eye Study	1992	4771	43 to 86	1.2
Rotterdam Study	1995	6251	55 to 98	1.1
Framingham Eye Study	1980	2631	Not defined	0.2 to 0.4
Third National Health and Nutrition Examination Survey	1995	4007	40+	0.4 including geographic atrophy
Baltimore Eye Study	1991	5308	40+	No prevalence neovascular AMD given
Chesapeake Bay Waterman Study	1989	777	30+	0.5

ed 5308 individuals in East Baltimore who were evaluated and diagnosed by screening ophthalmologists. The prevalence of AMD was 0.32% in white patients between the ages of 70 to 79 years, increasing to 2.9% in white individuals 80 years of age or older.[10] AMD was not formally defined by the study. The Beaver Dam Eye Study defined early AMD as drusen, RPE degeneration, or increased retinal pigmentation.[1] In patients aged 43 to 86 years, soft drusen were identified in 20.0% of eyes with pigmentary abnormalities in 13.1% of eyes.

Late age-related maculopathy (ARM) was defined as exudative AMD or geographic atrophy. Exudative changes were present in 1.2% with geographic atrophy occurring in 0.6% of the 4771 people examined.[1] A separate publication from the Beaver Dam Eye Study reported the 5-year incidence of late ARM. Exudative macular degeneration developed in at least one eye in 0.6% of the population and pure geographic atrophy developed in 0.3%.[4] The Rotterdam Study from the Netherlands evaluated 6251 individuals who were 55 to 98 years of age. Neovascular AMD occurred in 1.1% of the population with atrophic (geographic) AMD present in 0.6% of the evaluated population.[9] The Framingham Eye Study evaluated 5262 eyes and defined AMD (referred to as senile macular degeneration) as macular drusen, pigment disturbance, PED, or perimacular circinate exudates in an eye with 20/30 vision or worse. Dry AMD, consisting of macular drusen or pigment disturbance without exudation of fluid or subretinal fibrosis, occurred in 3.2% of eyes. Exudative AMD, defined as fluid or scar tissue beneath the macular retina, was present in 0.2% of eyes.[3] The Chesapeake Bay Waterman Study evaluated the fundus photographs of 777 male watermen over age 30 living along the eastern shore of Maryland. AMD was divided into exudative, nonexudative, and geographic atrophy. Eighty-five percent had one or more drusen in the macula, while only 0.5% was identified with exudative macular degeneration.[11]

PATHOPHYSIOLOGY OF AGE-RELATED MACULAR DEGENERATION

The cause of AMD and the formation of CNV remain unknown. The main focus has been on the degeneration of RPE cells with the formation of drusen as the instigating factor. The RPE cells are physiologically linked with the general health and function of the rod and cone cells. Degeneration of the RPE cells leads to deterioration of the photoreceptors as well as the choriocapillaris. The formation of drusen and pigmentary changes also appears to be associated with the metabolic failure of the RPE.[5,12]

RPE cells are involved in the daily enzymatic degradation of the membranous material shed by rods and cones. In younger individuals, waste products produced by the RPE are predominantly cleared by the choroid. Fluid is pumped from the retina into the choroid by healthy RPE cells, and nutrients diffuse from the choroid through the RPE to the retina.[12] In older individuals, abnormalities in the enzymatic process lead to the accumulation of molecular byproducts in the RPE cells, termed *residual bodies* or *lipofuscin granules*. Engorgement of RPE cells with residual bodies appears to interfere with their normal cellular metabolism. It is postulated that the deterioration of the RPE cells leads to extracellular excretions and deposits called drusen.[5,7] The defective enzymes determine the exact chemical composition of the material discharged from the RPE cells. Lipids in the basal deposits and drusen are assumed to be the result of failure of the RPE to process the cellular debris associated with the outer segment turnover and are deposited in Bruch's membrane.[12] It is believed that the deposition of lipid-rich material in Bruch's membrane produces a hydrophobic barrier that impedes the passage of fluid from the retina to the choroid, producing a detachment of the RPE. This hydrophobic barrier may also act to prohibit the movement of nutrients from the choroidal circulation to the RPE and retina.[12] The exact mechanism by which drusen incite choroidal vessels to abnormally grow is yet to be determined. CNV is felt to grow into the retina through breaks in Bruch's membrane.

A more recent approach by Friedman to the pathophysiology of AMD proposes that the etiology is a vascular disorder with hemodynamic alterations occurring secondary to atherosclerotic changes in the ocular vasculature.[13] Atherosclerosis occurs in older individuals and is defined as damage to the intimal layer of the vascular endothelium with lipid and cholesterol deposition.[14] The vessel wall becomes progressively thickened and less compliant. Normal aging also produces thickening of the sclera and Bruch's membrane.[12,15] The combination of increased ocular rigidity and decreased compliance of the vasculature supplying the eye increases the post-capillary resistance[16] and decreases the choroidal blood flow.[16-18] Hydrostatic pressure in the choriocapillaris increases with the elevation of post-capillary resistance, promoting exudation of extracellular proteins and lipids into the macula. The lipid exudates in Bruch's membrane take the form of basal deposits and drusen, ultimately leading to changes in the RPE that are seen with nonexudative AMD. The combination of drusen along with the degeneration of elastin and collagen causes calcification and fragmentation of Bruch's membrane. Neovascular AMD is induced from a combination of elevated choriocapillaris pressure, vascular endothelial growth factor induced by relative ischemia in the macula, and breaks in a calcified Bruch's membrane.

Friedman's model differs from the standard philosophy that the initial event in AMD is dysfunction of the RPE cells leading to deposition of drusen. Instead, Friedman's vascular model proposes that the RPE changes occur secondary to the deposition of lipid in Bruch's membrane.

Diminished ocular circulation between AMD and non-AMD eyes has been documented in many studies. Friedman et al[16] measured blood flow velocity and vessel pulsatility with color Doppler imaging. In patients with AMD, the pulsatility of arteries supplying the eye was higher with a decrease in blood flow velocity. This suggests an increased arteriolar resistance consistent with the hemodynamic model of the pathogenesis of AMD.

Ciulla et al[17] evaluated ocular blood flow velocities and the resistive index in retrobulbar vessels using color Doppler imaging in 25 patients with nonexudative AMD compared to 25 age-matched controls. Eyes with nonexudative AMD demonstrated a trend toward lower peak systolic and end diastolic velocities in the posterior ciliary arteries. End diastolic velocity of the nasal posterior ciliary artery was 26% less and represented the largest difference of the arteries tested. There was no significant difference in the resistive index of the posterior ciliary arteries. No difference between blood flow velocity and resistive index was identified in the ophthalmic artery. End diastolic velocity and the resistive index were significantly lower in the central retinal artery in the AMD group. These results imply that the choroidal perfusion is abnormal in AMD, and that changes in the central retinal artery imply a more generalized perfusion abnormality.[17]

Grunwald et al[18] evaluated the choroidal blood velocity and flow in the center of the fovea using laser Doppler flowmetry. Twenty subjects matched for age, intraocular pressure, and blood pressure with non-neovascular AMD and visual acuity of 20/32 or better were compared with 10 eyes without AMD. Choroidal blood volume was 33% lower and choroidal blood flow was 37% lower in the individuals with nonexudative AMD compared to normal controls.

NATURAL HISTORY OF SUBFOVEAL CHOROIDAL NEOVASCULARIZATION

Occult Choroidal Neovascularization

Natural history studies of occult CNV (Table 1-2) demonstrate that significant visual loss occurs with these lesions (see Figure 1-6). Bressler et al[19] retrospectively reviewed 84 eyes with occult CNV and reported that 63% lost 3 or more lines of vision with an average of 28

TABLE 1-2

NATURAL HISTORY OF OCCULT CHOROIDAL NEOVASCULARIZATION

1. Bressler et al:[19] 63% lost 3 or more lines over 28 months (84 eyes)
2. Stevens et al:[20] 29% lost 6 or more lines over 12 months (21 eyes)
3. MPS:[21] 41% lost 6 or more lines at 12 months, 64% lost 6 or more lines at 36 months (26 eyes)
4. RAD Study:[22] Mean decrease of 3.4 lines of visual acuity at 12 months (59 patients)

MPS = Macular Photocoagulation Study
RAD = Radiation for Age-Related Macular Degeneration

months of follow-up. The average visual acuity declined from an initial measurement of 20/80 to 20/250 during the same time period. Stevens et al[20] prospectively followed 21 eyes with occult CNV over a 12-month period and reported that 29% lost 6 or more lines of vision. The Macular Photocoagulation Study (MPS) Group[21] observed 26 eyes with occult CNV. Severe visual loss, consisting of a decrease in visual acuity of 6 or more lines of acuity, occurred in 41% of eyes at 12 months and 64% at 36 months. The median visual acuity at the 36-month point declined to 20/200 in the untreated eyes with occult CNV from an initial acuity of 20/50. Fifty-nine patients with occult CNV were followed as a control group in the Radiation Therapy for Age-Related Macular Degeneration Study Group. A mean of 3.4 lines of visual acuity were lost at 1 year.[22]

The Verteporfin in Photodynamic Therapy (VIP) Study Group followed 93 eyes with occult but no classic neovascularization in the placebo arm of the trial. At 12 months, 73% of these eyes experienced a loss of visual acuity from baseline, with 32% losing 6 or more lines. Two-year results of untreated eyes in the placebo group demonstrated 79% of eyes losing vision from baseline with 43% experiencing a decrease of 6 lines or more. Comparing the 1- and 2-year results of untreated occult lesions, a mean of 4 lines of visual acuity were lost at 12 months and 5 lines at 24 months after randomization. The average final visual acuity at 2 years was 20/160.[28]

Classic Choroidal Neovascularization

The MPS evaluated primary subfoveal CNV in a randomized trial commencing in 1986. Lesions were well demarcated, predominantly classic, occurring under the geometric center of the foveal avascular zone (FAZ) without prior laser treatment, and a maximum lesion size of 3.5 MPS disc areas. The control group served to define the natural history of well-defined, classic CNV. One hundred eighty-four patients in the no treatment group were initially followed with 63% receiving a 24-month examination.[23] Three months after randomization, the mean visual acuity in untreated eyes was 20/200, declining to 20/400 at 24 months. Visual acuity in untreated eyes decreased an average of 1.9 lines at 3 months and 4.4 lines at 24 months. Eleven percent had a decline of 6 or more lines of vision at 3 months. Thirty-seven percent of 112 untreated eyes examined at 24 months experienced the same decline of 6 or more lines.[23]

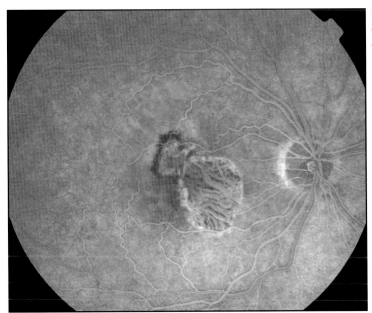

Figure 1-7. Recurrent CNV from a laser photocoagulation scar.

The MPS further evaluated recurrent subfoveal CNV at the edge of a scar (Figure 1-7) from laser treatment of extra- and juxtafoveal CNV secondary to AMD, ocular histoplasmosis, or idiopathic CNV due to high recurrence rates.[24,25] Fifty-two percent of laser-treated eyes with CNV secondary to AMD and 28% of laser-treated eyes with idiopathic or ocular histoplasmosis-induced CNV experienced subfoveal recurrences by 24 months.[25] One hundred nine eyes with well-demarcated CNV under the geometric center of the FAZ contiguous with scar from prior laser treatment were assigned to the observation group. The qualifying CNV lesion size was estimated on the final treatment scar (prior treatment scar and estimated newly treated area), which would be no larger than 6 disc areas and spare some retina within 1500 microns of the center of the FAZ.[26] The average visual acuity of the control eyes at study entry was 20/125. Three months following randomization, the average visual acuity decreased by 2 lines to 20/200. Forty-eight months after randomization, untreated eyes on average declined a total of 4 lines to 20/320.[24]

The Treatment of Age-Related Macular Degeneration with Photodynamic Therapy (TAP) Study Group also used an untreated control group to evaluate the efficacy of verteporfin, a photosensitizing agent, for the treatment of primary or recurrent subfoveal CNV.[27] Eligible lesions measured 5400 microns or less in greatest linear dimension with evidence of classic CNV and visual acuity 20/40 to 20/200. The control group consisted of 207 eyes. At 3 months, the average visual acuity was 20/126, declining to 20/200 at 12 months. The mean visual acuity remained stable at 20/200 at the 24-month examination. The observation group experienced a mean loss of 2 lines at 3 months, a mean of 3.5 lines of visual acuity at the 12-month follow-up examination, and 3.9 lines at the 24-month follow-up examination.

REFERENCES

1. Klein R, Klein BE, Linton KL. Prevalence of age-related maculopathy: the Beaver Dam Eye Study. *Ophthalmology.* 1992;99:933-943.

2. Munoz B, West SK, Rubin GS, et al. Causes of blindness and visual impairment in a population of older Americans: the Salisbury Eye Evaluation Study. *Arch Ophthalmol.* 2000;118:819-825.

3. Leibowitz HM, Krueger DE, Maunder LR, et al. The Framingham Eye Study Monograph: VI. Macular degeneration. *Surv Ophthalmol.* 1980;24(Suppl):428-457.

4. Klein R, Klein BE, Jensen SC, Meuer SM. The five-year incidence and progression of age-related maculopathy: the Beaver Dam Eye Study. *Ophthalmology.* 1997;104:7-21.

5. Young RW. Pathophysiology of age-related macular degeneration. *Surv Ophthalmol.* 1987;31:291-306.

6. Bressler SB, Rosberger DF. Non-neovascular (nonexudative) age-related macular degeneration. In: Guyer D, et al, eds. *Retina, Vitreous, Macula.* Philadelphia, Pa: WB Saunders; 1999.

7. Gass JDM. *Stereoscopic Atlas of Macular Diseases: Diagnosis and Treatment.* St. Louis, Mo: Mosby; 1997.

8. Lowenstein A, Bressler NM. Neovascular (exudative) age-related macular degeneration. In: Guyer D, et al, eds. *Retina, Vitreous, Macula.* Philadelphia, Pa: WB Saunders; 1999.

9. Vingerling JR, Dielemans I, Hofman A, et al. The prevalence of age-related maculopathy in the Rotterdam study. *Ophthalmology.* 1995;102:205-210.

10. Sommer A, Tielsch JM, Katz J, et al. Racial differences in cause-specific prevalence of blindness in East Baltimore. *N Engl J Med.* 1991;325:1412-1417.

11. Bressler NM, Bressler SB, West SK, et al. The grading and prevalence of macular degeneration in Chesapeake Bay watermen. *Arch Ophthalmol.* 1989;107:847-852.

12. Pauleikhoff D, Harper CA, Marshall J, Bird AC. Aging changes in Bruch's membrane: a histochemical and morphological study. *Ophthalmology.* 1990;97:171-178.

13. Friedman E. The role of the atherosclerotic process in the pathogenesis of age-related macular degeneration (editorial). *Am J Ophthalmol.* 2000;130:658-663.

14. Blood vessels. In: Cotran RS, Kumar V, Robbins SL, eds. *Robbins Pathologic Basis of Disease.* Philadelphia, Pa: WB Saunders; 1989:553-595.

15. Friedman E, Ivry M, Ebert E, et al. Increased scleral rigidity and age-related macular degeneration. *Ophthalmology.* 1989;96:104-108.

16. Friedman E, Krupsky S, Lane A, et al. Ocular blood flow velocity in age-related macular degeneration. *Ophthalmology.* 1995;102:640-646.

17. Ciulla T, Harris A, Chung HS, et al. Color Doppler imaging discloses reduced ocular blood flow velocities in nonexudative age-related macular degeneration. *Am J Ophthalmol.* 1999;128:75-80.

18. Grunwald JE, Hariprasad SM, DuPont J, et al. Foveolar choroidal blood flow in age-related macular degeneration. *Invest Ophthalmol Vis Sci.* 1998;39:385-390.

19. Bressler NM, Frost LA, Bressler SB, et al. Natural course of poorly defined choroidal neovascularization associated with macular degeneration. *Arch Ophthalmol.* 1988;106:1537-1542.

20. Stevens TS, Bressler NM, Maguire MG, et al. Occult choroidal neovascularization in age-related macular degeneration. A natural history study. *Arch Ophthalmol.* 1997;115:345-350.

21. Macular Photocoagulation Study Group. Occult choroidal neovascularization. Influence on visual outcome in patients with age-related macular degeneration. *Arch Ophthalmol.* 1996;114:400-412.

22. The Radiation Therapy for Age-Related Macular Degeneration Study Group. A prospective, randomized, double-masked trial on radiation therapy for neovascular age-related macular degeneration (RAD Study). *Ophthalmology.* 1999;106:2239-2247.

23. Macular Photocoagulation Study Group. Laser photocoagulation of subfoveal neovascular lesions in age-related macular degeneration: results of a randomized clinical trial. *Arch Ophthalmol.* 1991;109:1220-1231.

24. Macular Photocoagulation Study Group. Laser photocoagulation of subfoveal recurrent neovascular lesions in age-related macular degeneration: results of a randomized clinical trial. *Arch Ophthalmol.* 1991;109:1232-1241.

25. Macular Photocoagulation Study Group. Recurrent choroidal neovascularization after argon laser photocoagulation for neovascular maculopathy. *Arch Ophthalmol.* 1986;104:503-512.

26. Macular Photocoagulation Study Group. Subfoveal neovascular lesions in age-related macular degeneration: guidelines for evaluation and treatment in the macular photocoagulation study. *Arch Ophthalmol.* 1991;109:1242-1257.

27. Treatment of Age-Related Macular Degeneration with Photodynamic Therapy Study Group. Photodynamic therapy of subfoveal choroidal neovascularization in age-related macular degeneration with verteporfin. *Arch Ophthalmol.* 1999;117:1329-1345.

28. Verteporfin in Photodynamic Therapy Study Group. Photodynamic therapy of subfoveal choroidal neovascularization in age-related macular degeneration with verteporfin: 2-year results of a randomized clinical trial including lesions with occult but no classic neovascularization—VIP Report #2. *Am J Ophthalmol.* 2001;131:541-560.

CHAPTER TWO

SUBFOVEAL CHOROIDAL NEOVASCULARIZATION IN NON-AGE-RELATED MACULAR DEGENERATION

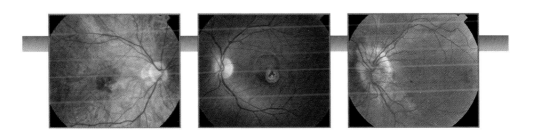

CHAPTER SECTIONS

INTRODUCTION

This chapter reviews the natural history and treatment outcomes of subfoveal choroidal neovascularization (CNV) in ocular histoplasmosis syndrome (OHS), idiopathic cases, pathologic myopia, and angioid streaks. In these conditions, subfoveal CNV generally impacts patients under the age of 50 and is not amenable to thermal laser photocoagulation. Aside from observation, the two primary treatment options are photodynamic therapy (PDT), which will be reviewed in Chapter Six, and submacular surgery. Submacular surgery is an attractive option in these patients since they typically have well-defined CNV located in the subretinal space anterior to the retinal pigment epithelium (RPE). These anatomical characteristics may allow the surgeon to remove the membrane with minimal damage to the RPE and choriocapillaris.[1] Case selection is greatly facilitated by imaging modalities, such as optical coherence tomography, that can accurately confirm the location of choroidal neovascular complexes in the subretinal space.[2,3] To date, studies of submacular surgery in non-age-related macular degeneration-related CNV have been small or retrospective and their results must be weighed accordingly. Until more definitive conclusions are available from the Submacular Surgery Trial (SST), a thorough understanding of these studies and their limitations (Tables 2-1 through 2-4) will enable the clinician to more effectively manage young patients with subfoveal CNV.

OCULAR HISTOPLASMOSIS SYNDROME

OHS is a common cause of CNV in young adults. The classic clinical triad for OHS includes CNV, peripapillary atrophy, and peripheral "punched-out" chorioretinal lesions or "histo spots."[4,5] OHS is also characterized by the absence of vitreal inflammation. The fungus *Histoplasma capsulatum* has been implicated as the etiologic agent for OHS based on positive skin testing and activation of the chorioretinal lesions on exposure to the histoplasmin antigen. The most important evidence, however, is epidemiological:[6-10]

- The highest prevalence of OHS occurs in areas where *Histoplasma capsulatum* is endemic, such as the Ohio and Mississippi river valleys
- OHS is rare outside endemic areas
- Most OHS patients live in or have previously lived in one of these endemic areas
- Greater than 90% of OHS patients have positive skin tests for *Histoplasma capsulatum*

While the organism has been identified in eyes from patients with disseminated histoplasmosis, it has never been cultured from or histopathologically observed in a patient with OHS.[11-13] The presence of human leukocyte antigen (HLA) markers B7, DR2, and DQ1 may genetically predispose individuals to OHS.[14-16] Myopic individuals with OHS may also be at higher risk of developing CNV.[17]

CNV from OHS usually impacts adults in the third and fourth decades of life.[18] Lewis and coworkers found the average age of symptomatic OHS was 40 years in first eyes and 44 years in second eyes.[19] In one endemic area, the prevalence of OHS was 4.4% and the prevalence of macular disciform scarring was 0.1%.[7] While OHS is much less prevalent in African-Americans, they are still at risk for significant visual loss secondary to macular disciform scarring.[20]

Natural History

There is a significant risk for visual loss in OHS patients with subfoveal CNV. Sixty-

TABLE 2-1

Natural History of Choroidal Neovascularization*

Diagnosis	Study	Study Size	Age	% Subfoveal CNV	Baseline VA <20/200	Final VA <20/200	Follow-Up (months)
OHS	Gass (1972)	14		100%		86%	Mean 36
	Klein (1977)	12		100%		67%	Mean 42
	Olk (1984)	66	Range 18-66	100%	58%	76%	Mean 42
	Kleiner (1988)	74	Median 45	100%	34% <20/100	77% <20/100	Median 36.5
Myopia	Hotchkiss (1981)+	27	Mean 45	51%	22%**	44%**	Mean 26
	Hampton (1983)	42	Range 12-96	58%	26%**	60%	Range <3 to >24
	Avila (1984)	70	Mean 52		57%	57%	Mean 41
	Tabandeh (1999)	22	Mean 63	55%	53%	73%	Mean 49
Idiopathic	VIP (2001)	39	Median 46	100%	None	26%	All eyes 12
	Ho (1995)	19	Mean 32	100%	26%	26%	Mean 88
Angioid streaks	Piro (1983)	33				50%	Range 1 to 168

*Table adapted in part from Tabandeh (1999)[44]
**Estimated from scattergram
+Six eyes (22%) had received prior laser photocoagulation
VIP = Verteporfin in Photocoagulation Therapy

TABLE 2-2

SUBMACULAR SURGICAL RESULTS*

Diagnosis	Study	Study Size (eyes)	Age	Baseline VA <20/200	Final VA <20/200	Follow-Up (months)	Recurrent CNV
OHS	Thomas (1994)	67	Median 42	48%	48%	Mean 10.5	37%
	Holekamp (1997)	117	Median 42	55%**	22%**	Median 13	44%
	Berger (1997)	63	Median 42	81%	63%	Median 24	38%
Myopia	Thomas (1994)	10	Median 39	30%	40%	Mean 7	20%
	Adelberg (1995)	5	Mean 44	60%	80%	Mean 11.5	20%
	Bottini (1996)	21	Median 53	81%	62%	Median 12	19%
	Uemura (2000)	23	Median 41	31%	48%	Mean 24	57%
Idiopathic	Thomas (1994)	8	Mean 40	100%	50%	Mean 6	50%
	Adelberg (1995)	4	Mean 41	100%	75%	Mean 18	50%
	Bottini (1996)	6	Median 49	50%	33%	Median 18	33%
Angioid	Thomas (1994)	4		100%	100%	Mean 7	25%
streaks	Adelberg (1995)	5	Mean 47	80%	80%	Mean 19	0%

*All studies included eyes with prior photocoagulation except Bottini (1996)
**Estimated from scattergram

TABLE 2-3

NATURAL HISTORY OF CHOROIDAL NEOVASCULARIZATION: PREDICTORS OF VISUAL OUTCOME

Diagnosis	Study	Positive Predictors	Negative Predictors
OHS	Olk (1984)	Age <40; extent of CNV <200 microns from FAZ center	Initial VA <20/200 >50% FAZ involved
	Kleiner (1988)	Age <30; small CNV complex; normal VA fellow eye	>50% FAZ involved
Myopia	Hampton (1983)		Age >30; CNV >400 microns in size
Idiopathic	Ho (1995)		CNV >1 DA

FAZ = foveal avascular zone

VA = visual acuity

DA = disc area

TABLE 2-4

SUBMACULAR SURGERY: PREDICTORS OF VISUAL OUTCOME

Diagnosis	Study	Positive Predictors	Negative Predictors
OHS	Thomas (1994)	Preop VA >20/100	
	Holekamp (1997)	Preop VA >20/100	Surgical complications
	Berger (1997)	Age <39	Recurrent CNV; preop laser treatment
Myopia	Bottini (1996)	Mean VA**	
	Uemura (2000)	Age >40*; recurrent	CNV*

*Trends only; study size was too small for statistical significance
**Mean VA = ([initial VA + final VA]/2)

seven to 86% of these eyes will have a final visual acuity of 20/200 or worse.[9,21-23] Spontaneous involution of CNV with a final visual acuity of 20/40 or better has been reported in up to 14% eyes with OHS and subfoveal CNV.[22] More favorable visual outcomes have been found in patients with younger ages, better initial visual acuities, and smaller neovascular complexes with a surrounding ring of pigmentation.[21-25] This pigmentation is often evident as a dark rim of hypofluorescence on fluorescein and indocyanine green angiography.[24,25] The risk of developing macular CNV in fellow eyes is 20% to 25%.[9,19,26-28] The Macular Photocoagulation Study (MPS) Group found a 2% incidence per year of CNV in fellow eyes of OHS patients with juxtafoveal or extrafoveal CNV after 5 years of follow-up[29]; 8% of patients with bilateral CNV were legally blind. The average time interval between CNV in first and second eyes is 4 years.[19] The presence of macular histo spots is the most significant risk factor for the development of CNV in fellow eyes.[6,9,29,30] Recurrent CNV after laser photocoagulation for juxtafoveal or extrafoveal CNV can be problematic: 40% of persistent or recurrent CNV in OHS patients in the MPS was subfoveal;[31] the median visual acuity in these patients was 20/125.

Treatment

Treatment of subfoveal CNV in OHS is challenging. Anecdotal reports have suggested that corticosteroids may be beneficial for treatment of CNV in OHS,[32] but no prospective, controlled studies have verified these findings. A small pilot study of thermal laser photocoagulation of subfoveal CNV had equivocal results and was discontinued due to low enrollment.[33] Due to its location anterior to the RPE, subfoveal CNV in OHS may be amenable to surgical removal.[1] Thomas and coworkers reported results of surgical removal of subfoveal CNV in 67 eyes with OHS.[34] Mean follow-up time was 10.5 months. Preoperative visual acuity was 20/200 or worse in 48% of eyes. Thirty-nine percent of eyes received prior laser treatment. Postoperatively, 48% of eyes had vision 20/200 or worse. The mean visual improvement was 1.4 Snellen lines. Visual acuity was 20/40 or better in 31% of eyes. Recurrent CNV occurred in 37% of eyes; in eyes followed for 12 months or more, the rate increased to 46%. Recurrence did not have a significant effect on visual outcome. Surgical complications occurred in 16% of eyes, including retinal detachment in four eyes and macular pucker in one eye. A follow-up study by the same group reported on surgical outcomes of 117 consecutive eyes with POHS and subfoveal CNV.[35] After a median follow-up time of 13 months, the mean visual improvement was 3 lines of visual acuity. Preoperative visual acuity was significantly correlated with visual outcome. Forty-four percent of eyes with a visual acuity of 20/100 or better obtained a postoperative visual acuity of 20/40 or better; in contrast, 25% of eyes with preoperative visual acuity of 20/200 or worse obtained a visual acuity of 20/40 or better. Recurrent CNV developed in 44% of eyes and, similar to their earlier study,[34] was not significantly associated with a poorer visual outcome. Surgical complications developed in 14% of eyes. Another study reported surgical outcomes on 63 eyes with OHS and subfoveal CNV followed for a median of 24 months.[36] Preoperatively, 81% of eyes had visual acuity of 20/200 or worse; mean visual acuity was 20/200. Fifty-one percent of eyes had received prior laser surgery. Postoperatively, 63% of eyes had visual acuity of 20/200 or worse. Mean visual acuity was 20/200; 35% of eyes improved by 2 or more lines of visual acuity. Factors correlated with improved visual prognosis included younger age, the lack of prior laser photocoagulation, and, unlike previous studies, preoperative visual acuity of 20/200 or worse. There was a 38% CNV recurrence rate after surgery; 67% of cases were subfoveal, often necessitating additional surgery. In contrast to earlier studies,[34,35] most eyes with recurrent CNV had a poor visual prognosis. Three percent of patients developed a retinal detachment.

While encouraging when compared to natural history studies, these surgical results must be interpreted cautiously due to the lack of controls, short follow-up periods, and the risk of postoperative complications.[37] More conclusive evidence on the role of surgery in the man-

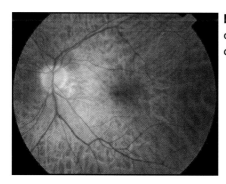

Figure 2-1. Pathologic myopia. There is a temporal crescent with thinning of the retina and prominent choroidal vasculature.

agement of subfoveal CNV in OHS will be forthcoming in the randomized, prospective, controlled multicenter submacular surgery trial (SST).[34]

PATHOLOGIC MYOPIA

Pathological myopia occurs in 2% of myopes[38] (Figure 2-1). The pathogenesis of pathologic myopia remains unclear, though genetic and environmental factors may both play a role. Pathologic myopia is characterized by excessive axial length with secondary degenerative changes in the sclera, choroid, Bruch's membrane, RPE, and retina. These changes are concentrated in the ora-equatorial zone and the posterior pole and typically occur in eyes with greater than 6 diopters of myopia and greater than 25 mm of axial length.[39] Ora-equatorial zone findings include "white without pressure," lattice degeneration, and pigmentary and paving-stone degeneration. Common posterior pole changes include optic nerve crescents, chorioretinal atrophy, lacquer cracks, and posterior staphyloma.[40,41] Posterior staphyloma is an important cause of blindness in pathologic myopes[42,43]; other vision-threatening complications include retinal detachment, chorioretinal atrophy, lacquer cracks, and CNV.

CNV occurs in 5% to 10% of patients with pathologic myopia and is subfoveal in greater than 50% of cases[40,41,44] (Figures 2-2 through 2-6). Linear breaks in Bruch's membrane secondary to stretching and degeneration of the choroid may place these eyes at risk for CNV. These breaks often appear clinically as lacquer cracks. Lacquer cracks have been associated with CNV in 82% of eyes with pathologic myopia[42]; microscopic defects in Bruch's membrane may be linked to CNV in eyes without lacquer cracks.[45] It is unclear, however, what causes the growth of CNV through the breaks in Bruch's membrane.[46] Quiescent CNV in myopes is often associated with a Fuchs' spot.[47]

Over 95% of CNV in pathologic myopes demonstrates mild hyperfluorescence confined to the early transit phase of the angiogram with minimal leakage beyond the borders of the lesion.[42,43] This CNV generally develops into a small atrophic scar, often with a surrounding rim of pigmentation characteristic of a Fuchs' spot. Since this pattern of CNV occurs in eyes with advanced myopic degeneration, its growth may be limited by underlying circulatory disturbances in the choroid and choriocapillaris due to mechanical stretching. CNV associated with more widespread leakage on angiography and the development of exudative disciform changes typically occurs in eyes with mild myopic degeneration.[42,43]

Natural History

Most natural history studies of CNV in pathologic myopia have not been limited to subfoveal CNV; thus, results must be interpreted conservatively. One study followed 27 myopic

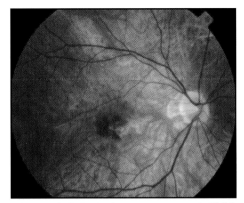

Figure 2-2. Pathologic myopia and CNV. Fine subretinal hemorrhage surrounds an area of hyperpigmentation in the fovea.

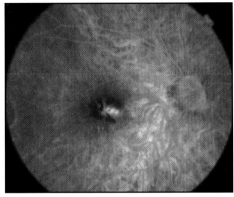

Figure 2-3. Late-phase angiogram of the same eye as in Figure 2-2 showing leakage from CNV confined to the area of pigmentation with minimal leakage beyond the border of the lesion.

Figure 2-4. Optical coherence tomography cross-section and map of the same eye as in Figures 2-2 and 2-3 demonstrating an increase in subretinal fluid from the actively leaking CNV.

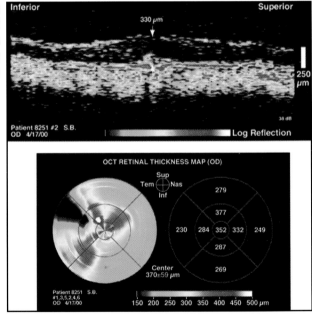

eyes with CNV for a mean of 25.5 months, including six that had received prior laser photocoagulation.[45] Fifty-one percent of eyes lost 2 or more lines of visual acuity compared to baseline; 44% progressed to 20/200 or worse. Hampton and coworkers followed 42 eyes with CNV, most of them for less than 2 years.[48] Fifty-eight percent had subfoveal CNV. Twenty-six percent had visual acuity of 20/200 or worse at baseline. They reported that 43% of eyes lost 2 or more lines of visual acuity and that 60% were left with 20/200 or worse visual acuity. Patients over 30 years of age had a poorer visual prognosis. Another study reported on 70 eyes with CNV followed for 41 months.[42] The CNV in the macula was not subclassified. The average age of the patients was 52 years. Fifty-seven percent had vision 20/200 or worse

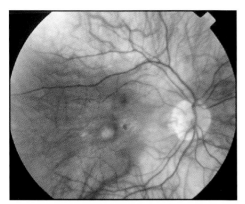

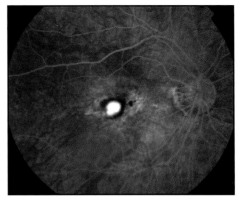

Figure 2-5. CNV in an eye with pathologic myopia. There is a temporal crescent adjacent to the optic nerve with thinning of the retina and prominent choroidal vasculature. The area of hyperpigmentation and retinal whitening corresponds to the CNV in Figure 2-6.

Figure 2-6. Late-phase angiogram showing leakage from CNV.

at baseline. Forty-six percent of eyes had decreased visual acuity from baseline; 57% had visual acuity of 20/200 or worse. However, poor visual acuity in the majority of cases was due to posterior staphylomas, not CNV; most of the eyes developed stable, nonexudative atrophic scars. An additional study followed 100 eyes with primarily juxtafoveal CNV for 5 years.[49] During the study period, all patients developed subfoveal CNV; their final visual acuity was 20/160. Older patients may have a poorer visual prognosis. In one study of 22 eyes with CNV and pathologic myopia, the average age of the patients was 63 years.[44] Fifty percent had vision of 20/200 or worse at baseline. Fifty-five percent of eyes had subfoveal CNV. At 1 year of follow-up, 73% had vision worse than 20/200, though 64% had the same or better vision at baseline.

One prospective natural history study of subfoveal CNV has been published from the Verteporfin in Photodynamic Therapy (VIP) Study Group.[50] This trial followed 39 patients with myopia and subfoveal CNV in its control group, which underwent sham treatment. The median age was 46 years. Baseline median visual acuity was 20/64. Only 5% of eyes had baseline visual acuity worse than 20/100. At 1 year of follow-up, 26% of eyes had a visual acuity of 20/160 or worse; their median visual acuity was 20/80. These encouraging outcomes are due in part to the very good baseline visual acuities of the VIP Study eyes. They may not be comparable to aforementioned natural history studies, which had much larger percentages of eyes with 20/200 or worse baseline visual acuity.

Treatment

Thermal laser photocoagulation of subfoveal CNV results in an immediate permanent decrease in vision with an absolute scotoma.[51] In pathologic myopes, the progressive enlargement of the laser scar can result in additional loss of visual acuity.[52] This knowledge, combined with the generally small atrophic scars that develop in myopes with CNV, has limited the value of laser photocoagulation in these patients.

Subretinal surgery may offer some visual benefits in pathologic myopes with subfoveal

CNV, especially those younger than 40 years of age. In one study, surgical removal of sub-foveal CNV was performed in 10 eyes with a mean follow-up of 7 months.[34] The median patient age was 39 years. Two eyes had received previous laser photocoagulation. Three eyes (30%) had a preoperative visual acuity of 20/200 or worse. The study reported a mean decrease of 1 line of preoperative visual acuity. Visual acuity was 20/200 or worse in four (40%) eyes. Two (20%) eyes had recurrent CNV. Adelberg and coworkers surgically removed subfoveal CNV in five eyes with pathologic myopia, four of which had received previous laser photocoagulation.[53] The mean age of the patients was 44 years; the mean follow-up time was 11.5 months. Three (60%) eyes had preoperative vision of 20/200 or worse. Four eyes (80%) had 20/200 or worse vision postoperatively. One eye had recurrent CNV. Another study examined surgical outcomes in 21 eyes with subfoveal CNV secondary to myopia for a median of 12 months.[54] None had previous laser treatment. The median age of the patients was 53. Eighty-one percent had preoperative vision worse than 20/200. Postoperatively, visual acuity stabilized or improved in 86% of eyes; visual acuity was 20/200 or worse in 62% of eyes. Nineteen percent of eyes had recurrent CNV. Ten percent of eyes had retinal detachments and 19% had cataract progression. An additional study examined surgical outcomes in 23 eyes with a mean follow-up of 24 months.[55] Thirty-one percent had preoperative vision of 20/200 or worse. Sixty-one percent had undergone previous laser photocoagulation. Visual acuity improved or stabilized in 65% of patients, with 48% of eyes left with a postoperative visual acuity of 20/200 or worse. Postoperative complications included retinal detachment (4%), endophthalmitis (4%), vitreous hemorrhage (4%), nuclear sclerotic cataracts (22%), and recurrent CNV (57%). Recurrent CNV was associated with a poorer prognosis. Age younger than 40 years was significantly correlated with improvement of 2 or more lines of vision after surgery.

It is difficult to assess the role of subretinal surgery in the management of patients with subfoveal CNV secondary to pathologic myopia. Most studies have been retrospective and uncontrolled and have included cases of recurrent as well as primary CNV. In addition, their results are not directly comparable to the VIP natural history data due to the poorer baseline visual acuities. Despite these drawbacks, subretinal surgery may be an option in patients younger than 40 years of age. Randomized, prospective controlled trials are needed to accurately assess the value of subretinal surgery in treating subfoveal CNV secondary to pathologic myopia. This would also facilitate comparison with outcomes from observation and photodynamic therapy in the VIP trial discussed in Chapter Six.

IDIOPATHIC CHOROIDAL NEOVASCULARIZATION

CNV in patients younger than 50 years of age often occurs secondary to degenerative changes, such as pathologic myopia or angioid streaks; inflammatory disease, such as ocular histoplasmosis or multifocal choroiditis; or trauma via choroidal rupture. Idiopathic CNV, however, occurs in this age group in otherwise healthy eyes[56] (Figures 2-7 through 2-10). The prevalence of idiopathic CNV in the United States is not known. However, a study in France—where OHS is not endemic—found that idiopathic CNV comprised 17% of all cases of CNV in patients younger than 50 years of age.[57] The average age of the patients was 37 years; 30% had subfoveal CNV. Ten percent of patients had bilateral CNV. The presence of both B7 and DR2 HLA markers may genetically predispose an individual to idiopathic CNV.[16] The relative risk for developing idiopathic CNV may also increase with diopters of myopia.[58]

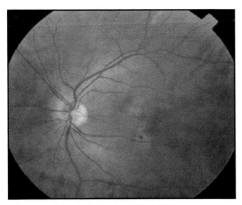

Figure 2-7. Idiopathic CNV. There are no other fundus findings revealing the etiology of the CNV.

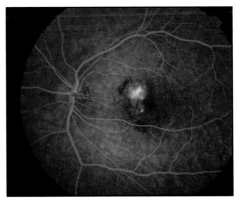

Figure 2-8. Late-phase angiogram of the eye in Figure 2-7 demonstrating leakage from CNV.

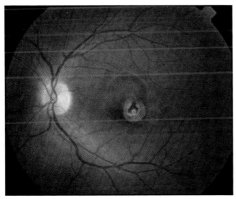

Figure 2-9. Recurrent idiopathic CNV after laser photocoagulation. Note the subretinal fluid superior to and surrounding the laser scar. Minimal subretinal hemorrhage exists at the edge of the scar and superior border of the neurosensory detachment.

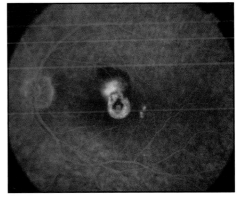

Figure 2-10. Late-phase angiogram of the eye in Figure 2-9 showing leakage from CNV and staining of the laser scar.

Natural History

While the natural history of idiopathic subfoveal CNV has not been studied prospectively, it may have a better prognosis than CNV secondary to AMD, myopia, or POHS. A retrospective study by Ho and coworkers[59] reported outcomes on 19 eyes with idiopathic CNV followed for an average of 88 months. The mean patient age was 32 years. The median initial visual acuity was 20/100; the median final visual acuity was 20/70. Thirty-one percent of patients had an initial visual acuity of 20/200 or worse; 31% of eyes had a final acuity of 20/200 or worse. Most significantly, 90% of patients improved or maintained their initial visual acuity. Age, sex, and initial visual acuity were not predictive of final visual acuity; CNV less than one disc area, though, was associated with a better visual outcome.

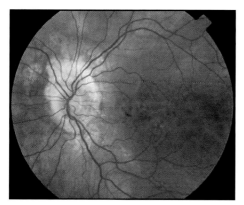

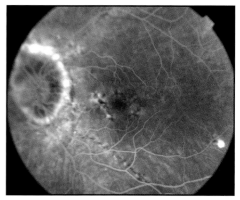

Figure 2-11. Angioid streaks with promi-nent peripapillary atrophy and light pig-mentation of the streak coursing through the macula. The angioid streaks are lightly pigmented and may be overlooked.

Figure 2-12. Fluorescein of the eye in Figure 2-11. The angioid streaks are stained by the fluorescein, making them more clearly defined.

Treatment

No treatment for subfoveal idiopathic CNV has been shown to be effective in a ran-domized, controlled clinical trial. However, several small retrospective studies on the use of submacular surgery to remove CNV in the subretinal space have demonstrated encouraging results.[1,52] In one study, eight eyes were followed for a mean of 6 months; three had received prior laser treatment.[34] Preoperative visual acuity was 20/200 or worse in all cases. Four (50%) eyes remained 20/200 or worse postoperatively; two (25%) had 20/40 or better visu-al acuity. Recurrent CNV developed in four (50%) cases. Another study followed four eyes for a mean of 18 months that underwent surgical removal of idiopathic subfoveal CNV.[53] Two eyes had high myopia. One eye had received prior laser treatment. All had 20/200 or worse visual acuity preoperatively. One eye improved to 20/25; the three remaining eyes remained 20/200 or worse postoperatively. One eye developed a retinal break. Bottoni and coworkers removed idiopathic CNV from six eyes and followed them for a median of 18 months.[54] Three (50%) eyes had preoperative visual acuity of 20/200 or worse. Postoperatively, two (33%) eyes had 20/200 or worse visual acuity and three had 20/40 or better visual acuity. Two (33%) eyes developed recurrent CNV. These studies must be inter-preted with caution, given their retrospective nature and small size. The definitive role of submacular surgery in the management of idiopathic CNV will be more clearly defined by the submacular surgery trials.[32]

ANGIOID STREAKS

Angioid streaks are visible linear, full-thickness breaks in Bruch's membrane that extend radially from the peripapillary area[60] (Figures 2-11 and 2-12). They typically appear in the second decade of life and are usually bilateral and symmetric. The color of the streaks depends upon fundus pigmentation, ranging from dark brown in heavily pigmented individ-uals to red in lightly pigmented individuals.[61] When the streaks atrophy, they take on a yel-low appearance. A mottled, *peau d'orange* fundus and optic disc drusen have also been asso-

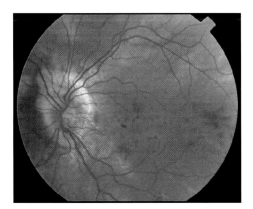

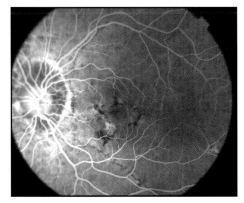

Figure 2-13. Extrafoveal subretinal hemorrhage along an angioid streak in the same eye as in Figures 2-11 and 2-12.

Figure 2-14. Fluorescein angiography of the eye in Figure 2-13. An extrafoveal CNV is visible adjacent to the subretinal hemorrhage.

ciated with angioid streaks.[62] This characteristic ophthalmoscopic appearance usually makes the diagnosis of angioid streaks straightforward; early in the disease, however, fluorescein and indocyanine green angiography may be helpful in revealing more subtle streaks and fundus mottling.[63-67]

The pathogenesis of angioid streaks is unknown. Histopathologically, there is evidence of extensive calcium deposition in Bruch's membrane and breaks that correspond to the clinically observed angioid streaks.[61] There is also atrophy of the underlying choriocapillaris and overlying RPE.[68] The thickened and brittle Bruch's membrane may crack when subject to the routine stretching of the extraocular muscles (EOMs); the characteristic radial pattern of the streaks may arise because the base of the vector forces exerted by the EOMs is at the scleral foramen.[69] These cracks in Bruch's membrane place patients at high risk for the development of CNV.

Angioid streaks have been classically linked to systemic diseases such as pseudoxanthoma elasticum (PXE), Paget's disease, and sickle cell anemia, all of which have histopathological evidence of abnormal calcium deposition in Bruch's membrane.[70-72] PXE is the most common association, occurring in up to 60% of patients with angioid streaks.[73] Rarer systemic associations include Ehlers-Danlos disease, sickle-thalassemia, hereditary spherocytosis, and abetalipoproteinemia.[74,75] Idiopathic angioid streaks occur in 35% to 50% of patients.[69,76]

Visual outcomes are poor in patients with angioid streaks. In a group of 62 patients followed for a mean of 3.6 years, 50% were legally blind at their most recent follow-up visit.[76] Aside from traumatic retinal hemorrhage,[77-79] the most significant vision-threatening complication of angioid streaks is the development of CNV (Figures 2-13 and 2-14). CNV can occur in 72% to 86% of eyes with angioid streaks and is bilateral in 49% to 60% of cases.[60,76] The CNV is usually well-defined and in the immediate proximity of a streak. The risk of CNV increases with age. Patients with PXE are at high risk for CNV-induced visual loss in the third and fourth decades of life.[73] Clinical signs associated with CNV include the diffuse type of streaks, streaks longer than 3 disc diameters, and streaks passing through the fovea.[80]

There are few natural history studies of CNV in patients with angioid streaks. Piro and coworkers retrospectively reported on 33 eyes that presented with active CNV and were followed without treatment for a range of 1 month to 14 years.[76] While the subclassification of the CNV was not specified, 50% of eyes were legally blind at the time of their last examination. Laser treatment may not alter this course: in the same study, 11 patients were treated for extrafoveal lesions; 73% (8) were legally blind at the time of their last visit.

While recent studies suggest that eyes with extrafoveal CNV may benefit from laser photocoagulation, especially if MPS treatment criteria are rigidly adhered to with respect to intensity and extent of treatment,[81,82] there is no effective treatment for subfoveal CNV. Several small series have reported discouraging results with submacular surgery. Thomas and coworkers[34] reported on four eyes with subfoveal CNV secondary to angioid streaks followed for a mean of 7 months. Pre- and postoperative visual acuity was 20/200 or worse in all eyes. One eye developed recurrent CNV. Adelberg and coworkers[53] removed subfoveal CNVMs from five eyes with angioid streaks. The mean patient age was 47 years. The mean follow-up was 19 months. One eye had improvement of visual acuity from 20/300 to 20/50; the remaining eyes had postoperative vision worse than 20/200, including one eye that decreased from 20/80 to counting fingers. One eye developed a retinal detachment postoperatively. No recurrent CNV was reported.

CONCLUSION

While further studies of PDT and data from the SST will ultimately determine the impact of these treatment modalities on the natural history of subfoveal CNV, the following trends can be gleaned from the data to date (see Tables 2-1 through 2-4):

* OHS patients have poor visual outcomes if the CNV is untreated. More favorable results have occurred after surgical removal of the subfoveal CNV, especially in patients younger than 40 years with good visual acuity and no history of prior laser photocoagulation.
* Younger patients with pathologic myopia and good initial visual acuity have a better natural history than those with OHS; submacular surgery may be beneficial in patients with poorer visual acuity, especially patients older than 50 years.
* Untreated idiopathic cases have the most favorable visual outcomes compared to their counterparts with OHS, myopia, or angioid streaks; it is unclear whether submacular surgery results are better than the natural history of the disease.
* Patients with angioid streaks and CNV have poor visual outcomes regardless of observation or treatment. Results from photodynamic therapy and submacular surgery are only available in a small number of patients.

REFERENCES

1. Gass JDM. Biomicroscopic and histopathologic considerations regarding the feasibility of surgical excision of subfoveal neovascular membranes. *Am J Ophthalmol.* 1994;118:285-298.

2. Giovannini A, Amato GP, Mariotti C, et al. OCT imaging in choroidal neovascularization and its role in the determination of patient's eligibility for surgery. *Br J Ophthalmol.* 1999;83:438-442.

3. Iida T, Hagimura N, Sato T, et al. Optical coherence tomographic features of idiopathic submacular choroidal neovascularization. *Am J Ophthalmol.* 2000;130:763-768.

4. Woods AC, Whalen HE. The probable role of benign histoplasmosis in the etiology of granulomatous uveitis. *Trans Am Ophthalmol Soc.* 1959;57:318-343.

5. Schlaegel TF, Kenney D. Changes around the optic nerve head in presumed ocular histoplasmosis. *Am J Ophthalmol.* 1966;62:454-458.

6. Ellis FD, Schlaegel TF. The geographic localization of presumed ocular histoplasmosis choroiditis. *Am J Ophthalmol.* 1975;75:953-956.

7. Smith RE, Ganley JP. An epidemiological study of presumed ocular histoplasmosis. *Trans Am Acad Ophthalmol Otolaryngol.* 1971;75:994-1005.

8. Ganley JP. Epidemiologic characteristics of presumed ocular histoplasmosis. *Acta Ophthalmol Suppl.* 1973;119(Suppl):1-63.

9. Gass JDM, Wilkinson CP. Follow-up study of presumed ocular histoplasmosis syndrome. *Trans Am Acad Ophthalmol Otolaryngol.* 1972;75:994-1005.

10. Schlaegel TF. Granulomatous uveitis: an etiologic survey of 100 cases. *Trans Am Acad Ophthalmol Otolaryngol.* 1958;62:813-825.

11. Craig EL, Suie T. Histoplasma capsulatum in human ocular tissue. *Arch Ophthalmol.* 1974;91:285-280.

12. Klintworth GK, Hollingsworth AS, Lusman PA, Bradford WD. Granulomatous choroiditis in a case of disseminated histoplasmosis. *Arch Ophthalmol.* 1973;92:45-48.

13. Goldstein BG, Buettner H. Histoplasmic endophthalmitis. A clinicopathologic correlation. *Arch Ophthalmol.* 1983;101:774-777.

14. Braley RE, Meredith TA, Aaberg TM, et al. The prevalence of HLA-B7 in presumed ocular histoplasmosis. *Am J Ophthalmol.* 1978;85:859-861.

15. Godfrey WA, Cross DE, Ziemanski MC, et al. HLA-B7 in presumed ocular histoplasmosis. *Transplant Proc.* 1979;11:1874-1876.

16. Duqesnoy RJ, Annen K, Meredith TA. Association of presumed ocular histoplasmosis with HLA-B7 and DRw2. *Transplant Proc.* 1979;11:1877-1878.

17. Derosa JT, Yannussi LA, Marmor M, et al. Risk factors for choroidal neovascularization in young patients: a case-control study. *Documenta Ophtalmologica.* 1996;91:207-222.

18. Schlaegel TF. The natural history of spots in the disc-macula area. *Int Ophthalmol Clin.* 1975;15:19-28.

19. Lewis ML, Van Newkirk MR, Gass JDM. Follow-up of presumed ocular histoplasmosis syndrome. *Ophthalmology.* 1980;87:390-399.

20. Baskin MA, Jampol LM, Huamonte FU, et al. Macular lesions in blacks with the presumed ocular histoplasmosis syndrome. *Am J Ophthalmol.* 1980;89:77-83.

21. Kleiner RC, Enger C, Fine SL. Subfoveal neovascularization in the ocular histoplasmosis syndrome: a natural history study. *Retina.* 1988;8:225-229.

22. Olk RJ, Burgess DB, McCormick PA. Subfoveal and juxtafoveal subretinal neovascularization in the presumed ocular histoplasmosis syndrome. *Ophthalmology.* 1984;91:1592-1602.

23. Klein ML, Fine SL, Knox DL, et al. Follow-up study in eyes with choroidal neovascularization caused by presumed ocular histoplasmosis. *Am J Ophthalmol.* 1977;83:830-835.

24. Campochiaro PA, Morgan KM, Conway BP, Stathos J. Spontaneous involution of subfoveal neovascularization. *Am J Ophthalmol.* 1990;109:668-675.

25. Iida T, Hagimura N, Kishi S, et al. Indocyanine green angiographic features of idiopathic submacular choroidal neovascularization. *Am J Ophthalmol.* 1998;126:70-76.

26. Lewis ML, Schiffman JC. Long-term follow-up of the second eye in ocular histoplasmosis. *Int Ophthalmol Clin.* 1983;23:281-285.

27. Elliot JH, Jackson DJ. Presumed histoplasmic maculopathy: clinical course and prognosis in nonphotocoagulated eyes. *Int Ophthalmol Clin.* 1975;15:29-39.

28. Sawelson H, Goldberg RE, Annesley WH, Tomer TL. Presumed ocular histoplasmosis syndrome. The fellow eye. *Arch Ophthalmol.* 1976;94: 221-224.

29. Macular Photocoagulation Study Group. Five year follow-up of fellow eyes of individuals with ocular histoplasmosis and unilateral extrafoveal or juxtafoveal choroidal neovascularization. *Arch Ophthalmol.* 1996;114:677-688.

30. Feman SS, Podgorski SF, Penn MK. Blindness from presumed ocular histoplasmosis in Tennessee. *Ophthalmology.* 1982;89:1295-1298.

31. Macular Photocoagulation Study Group. Persistent and recurrent neovascularization after krypton laser photocoagulation for neovascular lesions of ocular histoplasmosis. *Arch Ophthalmol.* 1989;107:344-352.

32. Schlaegel TF. Corticosteroids in the treatment of ocular histoplasmosis. *Int Ophthalmol Clin.* 1993;23:111-123.

33. Fine SL, Wood WJ, Singerman LJ, et al. Laser treatment for subfoveal neovascular membranes in ocular histoplasmosis syndrome: results of a pilot randomized clinical trial. *Arch Ophthalmol.* 1993;111:19-20.

34. Thomas MA, Dickinson JD, Melberg NS, et al. Visual results after surgical removal of subfoveal choroidal neovascularization. *Ophthalmology.* 1994;101:1384-1396.

35. Holekamp NM, Thomas MA, Dickinson JD, et al. Surgical removal of subfoveal choroidal neovascularization in presumed ocular histoplasmosis. *Ophthalmology.* 1997;104:22-26.

36. Berger AS, Conway M, Del Priore LV, et al. Submacular surgery for subfoveal choroidal neovascularization membranes in patients with presumed ocular histoplasmosis. *Arch Ophthalmol.* 1997;115:991-996.

37. Bressler NM. Submacular surgery. New information, new questions. *Arch Ophthalmol.* 1997;115:1071-1072.

38. Michaels DD. *Visual Optics and Refraction. A Clinical Approach.* 2nd ed. St. Louis, Mo: CV Mosby; 1980:513.

39. Curtin BJ. Physiologic vs pathologic myopia: genetics vs environment. *Ophthalmology.* 1979;86:681-691.

40. Curtin BJ, Karlin DB. Axial length measurements and fundus changes of the myopic eye. *Am J Ophthalmol.* 1971;1:42-53.

41. Grossniklaus HE, Green WR. Pathologic findings in pathologic myopia. *Retina.* 1992;12:127-133.

42. Avila MP, Weiter JJ, Jalkh AE, et al. Natural history of choroidal neovascularization in degenerative myopia. *Ophthalmology.* 1984;91:1573-1581.

43. Jalkh AE, Weiter JJ, Trempe CL, et al. Choroidal neovascularization in degenerative myopia: role of laser photocoagulation. *Ophthalmic Surg.* 1987;18:721-725.

44. Tabandeh H, Flynn HW, Scott IU, et al. Visual acuity outcomes of patients 50 years of age and older with high myopia and untreated choroidal neovascularization. *Ophthalmology.* 1999;106:2063-2067.

45. Hotchkiss ML, Fine SL. Pathologic myopia and choroidal neovascularization. *Am J Ophthalmol.* 1981;91:177-183.

46. Fine SL. Discussion re: visual prognosis of disciform degeneration in myopia by Hampton GR, Kohen D, Bird AC. *Ophthalmology.* 1983;90:926.

47. Levy JH, Pollock HM, Curtain BJ. The Fuchs" spot: an ophthalmoscopic and fluorescein angiographic study. *Ann Ophthalmol.* 1977;9:1433-1343.

48. Hampton GR, Kohen D, Bird AC. Visual prognosis in disciform degeneration in myopia. *Ophthalmology.* 1983;90:923-926.

49. Secretan M, Kuhn D, Soubrane G, Coscas G. Long-term visual outcome of choroidal neovascularization in pathologic myopia: natural history and laser treatment. *Eur J Ophthalmol.* 1997;7:307-316.

50. Verteporfin in Photodynamic Therapy Study Group. Photodynamic therapy of subfoveal choroidal neovascularization in pathologic myopia with verteporfin: one year results of a randomized clinical trial—VIP report #1. *Ophthalmology.* 2001;108:841-852.

51. Macular Photocoagulation Study Group. Laser photocoagulation of subfoveal neovascular lesions in age-related macular degeneration: results of a randomized clinical trial. *Arch Ophthalmol.* 1991;109:1220-1231.

52. Brancato R, Pece A, Avanza P, Radrizzani. Photocoagulation scar expansion after laser therapy for choroidal neovascularization in degenerative myopia. *Retina.* 1990;10:239-243.

53. Adelberg DA, Del Priore LV, Kaplan HJ. Surgery for subfoveal membranes in myopia, angioid streaks and other disorders. *Retina.* 1995;15:198-205.

54. Bottoni F, Airaghi P, Perego E, et al. Surgical removal of idiopathic, myopic and age-related subfoveal neovascularization. *Graefe's Arch Clin Exp Ophthalmol.* 1996;234:S42-S50.

55. Uemura A, Thomas MA. Subretinal surgery for choroidal neovascularization in patients with high myopia. *Arch Ophthalmol.* 2000;118:44-350.

56. Cleasby GW. Idiopathic focal subretinal neovascularization. *Am J Ophthalmol.* 1976;81:590-596.

57. Cohen SY, Laroche A, Leguen Y. Etiology of choroidal neovascularization in young patients. *Ophthalmology.* 1996;103:1241-1244.

58. Spitznas M, Boker T. Idiopathic posterior subretinal neovascularization (ISPN) is related to myopia. *Graefe's Arch Clin Exp Ophthalmol.* 1991;229:536-538.

59. Ho AC, Yannuzzi LA, Pisicano K, et al. The natural history of idiopathic subfoveal choroidal neovascularization. *Ophthalmology.* 1995;102:782-789.

60. Shields JA, Federman JL, Tomer TL, et al. Angioid streaks I. Ophthalmic variations and diagnostic problems. *Br J Ophthalmol.* 1975;59:257-266.

61. Clarkson JG, Altman RD. Angioid streaks. *Surv Ophthalmol.* 1982;26:235-246.

62. Coleman K, Ross MH, Mc Cabe M, et al. Disc drusen and angioid streaks in pseudoxanthoma elasticum. *Am J Ophthalmol.* 1991;112:166-170.

63. Smith JL, Gass JDM, Justice J. Fluorescein fundus photography of angioid streaks. *Br J Ophthalmol.* 1964;48:517-521.

64. Quaranta M, Cohen SY, Krott R. Indocyanine green videoangiography of angioid streaks. *Am J Ophthalmol.* 1995;119:136-142.

65. Pece A, Avanza P, Introini U, Brancato R. Indocyanine green angiography in angioid streaks. *Acta Ophthalmol Scand.* 1997;75:261-265.

66. Lafaut BA, Leys AM, Scassellati-Sforzolini B, et al. Comparison of fluorescein and indocyanine green angiography in angioid streaks. *Graefe's Arch Clin Exp Ophthalmol.* 1998;236:346-353.

67. Mansour AM, Ansari NH, Shields JA, et al. Evolution of angioid streaks. *Ophthalmologica.* 1993;207:57-61.

68. Dreyer R, Green WR. The pathology of angioid streaks: a study of twenty-one cases. *Trans Pa Acad Ophthalmol Otolaryngol.* 1978;31:158-167.

69. Mansour AM. Systemic associations of angioid streaks. *Int Ophthalmol Clin.* 1991;31:61-68.

70. Paton D. Angioid streaks and sickle cell anemia: a report of two cases. *Arch Ophthalmol.* 1959;62:852-858.

71. Gass JDM, Clarkson JG. Angioid streaks and disciform macular detachment in Paget's disease (Osteitis deformans). *Am J Ophthalmol.* 1973;75:576-586.

72. Jampol LM, Acheson R, Eagle RC, et al. Calcification of Bruch's membrane in angioid streaks with homozygous sickle cell disease. *Arch Ophthalmol.* 1987;105:93-98.

73. Shilling JS, Blach RK. Prognosis and therapy of angioid streaks. *Br J Ophthalmol.* 1975;95:301-305.

74. Aessopos A, Voskaridou E, Kavouklis E, et al. Angioid streaks in sickle-thalassemia. *Am J Ophthalmol.* 1994;117:589-592.

75. McLane NJ, Grizzard S, Kousseff BG, et al. Angioid streaks associated with hereditary spherocytosis. *Am J Ophthalmol.* 1984;97:444-449.

76. Piro PA, Scherga D, Fine SL. Angioid streaks. Natural history and visual prognosis. In: Fine SL, Owens SL, eds. *Management of Retinal Vascular and Macular Disorders.* Baltimore, Md: Williams & Wilkins; 1983:136-139.

77. Hagedoorn A. Angioid streaks and traumatic ruptures of Bruch's membrane. *Br J Ophthalmol.* 1975;59:267.

78. Levin DB, Bell DK. Traumatic retinal hemorrhages with angioid streaks. *Arch Ophthalmol.* 1977;95:1072-1073.

79. Schneiderman TE, Kalina RE. Subretinal hemorrhage precedes development of angioid streaks. *Arch Ophthalmol.* 1994;112:1622-1623.

80. Mansour AM, Shields JA, Annesley WH, et al. Macular degeneration in angioid streaks. *Ophthalmologica.* 1988;197:36-41.

81. Gelisken O, Hendrikse F, Deutman AF. A long-term follow-up study of laser coagulation of neovascular membranes in angioid streaks. *Am J Ophthalmol.* 1988;105:299-303.

82. Lim JI, Bressler NM, Marsh MJ, Bressler SB. Laser treatment of choroidal neovascularization in patients with angioid streaks. *Am J Ophthalmol.* 1993;116:414-423.

CHAPTER THREE

DIAGNOSTIC IMAGING FOR PHOTODYNAMIC THERAPY: FLUORESCEIN ANGIOGRAPHY AND OPTICAL COHERENCE TOMOGRAPHY

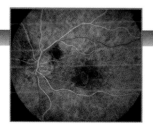 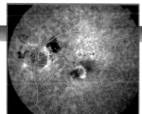 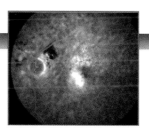

CHAPTER SECTIONS

FLUORESCEIN ANGIOGRAPHY OVERVIEW

Fluorescein angiography is currently the gold standard for the evaluation of age-related macular degeneration (AMD). It is also the diagnostic imaging modality used in major trials for the treatment of choroidal neovascularization, including the Macular Photocoagulation Study (MPS) and Treatment of Age-Related Macular Degeneration with Photodynamic Therapy (TAP) Study. These studies have emphasized the importance of identifying classic choroidal neovascularization (CNV) and differentiating it from other patterns of fluorescence.

A detailed discussion of the principles of fluorescein angiography is beyond the scope of this text. After sodium fluorescein is injected intravenously, 80% becomes protein-bound and the other 20% is available for fluorescence. The fluorescein is activated by blue light energy between 465 and 490 nm, resulting in fluorescence at a green-yellow wavelength of 520 to 530 nm. Filters on digital or film-based systems are used to isolate this fluorescence from the fundus and create an angiogram as the chemical circulates through the choroidal and retinal vasculature. Sodium fluorescein is able to diffuse through the choriocapillaris but is retained by intact retinal vascular endothelium and retinal pigment epithelium (RPE).

Patterns of hyperfluorescence include transmission defects, leakage, pooling, staining, and autofluorescence/pseudofluorescence. Each of these manifests as increased fluorescence following different time intervals and characteristics based on the causative pathology.

Transmission defects result from atrophy or diminished pigment in the RPE, allowing normal fluorescence from the underlying choriocapillaris to appear more intense (Figure 3-1). The timing of this hyperfluorescent pattern follows the filling and emptying of fluorescein from the choriocapillaris. This is characterized by early hyperfluorescence that fades late and maintains a constant size and shape determined by the structural RPE defect.

Leakage occurs when intravascular fluorescein exits normal vascular or tissue barriers. In the normal eye, the retinal vascular endothelium serves as a barrier to retinal vascular leakage and the RPE serves as a barrier to choroidal leakage. Specific types of leakage include pooling in distinct anatomic spaces or staining of fixed tissue structures such as drusen, fibrosis, or the sclera. Leakage patterns in CNV are reviewed below and show distinct characteristics. It is important to understand these patterns with respect to their structural and temporal characteristics in order to properly diagnose their etiology. Leakage into the subretinal space is the hallmark of classic CNV. Bright, uniform hyperfluorescence is noted early and increased fluorescence is noted in the later frames of the angiogram, when most of the intravascular fluorescence has faded (Figure 3-2). The borders of this abnormal fluorescence tend to expand late as a result of this leakage. In contrast, pooling of fluorescein in the sub-RPE space (eg, serous pigment epithelial detachment [PED]) tends to maintain fixed borders due to firm adherence of the RPE to Bruch's membrane (Figure 3-3). Staining of tissue structures also maintains fixed borders as determined by the tissue being stained.

Autofluorescence and pseudofluorescence occur prior to the injection of fluorescein. Autofluorescence is seen with structures that possess intrinsic fluorescence such as optic nerve head drusen and astrocytic hamartoma. Pseudofluorescence is a camera artifact caused by mismatched filters.

Hypofluorescence is caused by blockage or a perfusion-related filling defect. Blockage of fluorescence may be caused by anything that obstructs the transmission of fluorescence from the fundus to the camera (Figure 3-4). Common causes in AMD include hemorrhage, exudate, and pigment. Perfusion-related filling defects result from an obstruction or absence of vessels. After conventional laser photocoagulation, for example, the choriocapillaris is

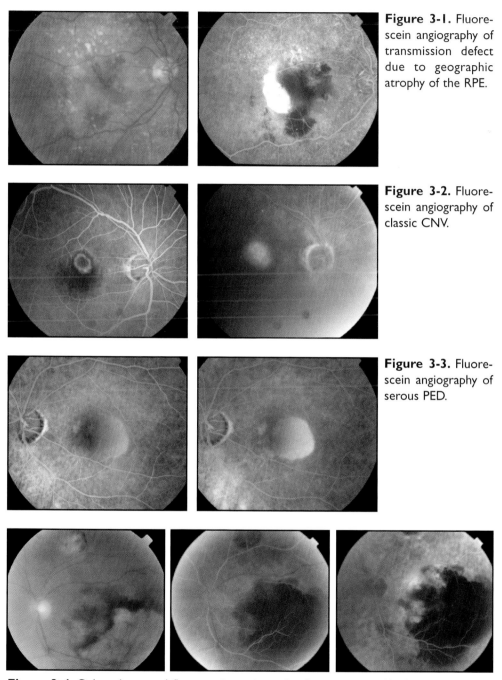

Figure 3-1. Fluorescein angiography of transmission defect due to geographic atrophy of the RPE.

Figure 3-2. Fluorescein angiography of classic CNV.

Figure 3-3. Fluorescein angiography of serous PED.

Figure 3-4. Color photo and fluorescein angiography demonstrating blockage by chronic, organized subretinal hemorrhage.

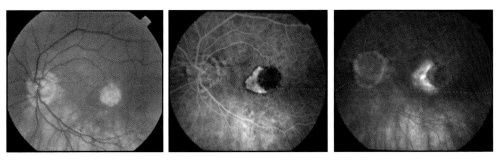

Figure 3-5. Color photo and fluorescein angiography showing hypofluorescent laser scar with hyperfluorescent, recurrent subfoveal CNV.

destroyed in the treated area and cannot fill with fluorescein from the circulation (Figure 3-5). As a result, a laser scar exhibits choroidal hypofluorescence (although staining of the sclera may occur at the borders from adjacent intact choriocapillaris).

Interpretation of angiographic patterns of fluorescence allows definitive classification of lesions into subtypes representing their anatomic and physiologic characteristics. This is important when considering treatment options since the various lesion types respond differently to currently available therapies.

OPTICAL COHERENCE TOMOGRAPHY OVERVIEW

Optical coherence tomography (OCT) is a noninvasive imaging modality capable of producing micron-resolution cross-sectional images of biological tissues.[1-4] OCT accurately represents specific structural characteristics of the retina and can provide objective anatomic measurements. The diagnostic information complements conventional imaging techniques such as fluorescein and indocyanine green angiography.

The mechanism of OCT is analogous to ultrasound B-mode imaging with several distinct advantages. The use of light instead of acoustic waves allows for spatial resolution in the 10 to 20 micron range, approximately 10 times higher than B-mode ultrasound. Traditional B-mode ultrasound, using a sound wave frequency of 10 megahertz, yields spatial resolutions of approximately 150 microns. In addition, the use of light allows an image to be obtained noninvasively, without direct contact to the globe. Cross-sectional images can be obtained rapidly in approximately 2.5 seconds.

A particularly useful application of OCT is in the localization, detection, and measurement of retinal fluid. A fluid collection is accurately depicted in its anatomic layer whether it be intraretinal, subretinal, or under the RPE. OCT can provide clinically useful information about neovascular AMD since it manifests by changing macular thickness or accumulation of fluid in the macula. It also has utility in following response to photodynamic therapy (PDT) and guiding retreatment decisions.

Interpretation of OCT images of AMD requires familiarity with the OCT representation of a normal posterior segment and knowledge of basic OCT principles. The strength of the OCT signal at a particular tissue layer is dependent on several factors. Signal strength is defined by the following:
- The amount of incident light transmitted to a particular layer without being absorbed by intervening tissue
- The amount of transmitted light that is backscattered

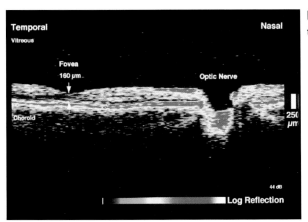

Figure 3-6. Normal OCT through the optic nerve and macula.

- The fraction of backscattered light that returns to the detector without being further attenuated

Reflectivity is the portion of incident light that is directly backscattered by a tissue. The OCT signal from any particular tissue layer is a function of its reflectivity and the absorption and scattering properties of the overlying tissue layers.[1] For example, a tissue with a high level of backscatter that lies deep to a tissue with low absorption and low backscatter will produce a high signal.

The signal strength can be represented in grayscale or as the false color representation used for the images that follow. Figure 3-6 shows an OCT image of a normal eye scanned through the optic nerve and macula. The vitreoretinal interface is characterized by a demarcation in contrast from the nonreflective vitreous and the highly reflective nerve fiber layer (NFL). High backscatter is represented by red-orange color and low backscatter appears blue-black. False color is represented by the normal visible spectrum. The fovea has a characteristic depression with thinning of the retina corresponding to its normal anatomy.

A bright red-orange layer that delineates the posterior boundary of the retina corresponds to the RPE and choriocapillaris. There is contrast between the less reflective photoreceptors and the highly backscattered RPE. The thin, dark layer anterior to the RPE layer represents the photoreceptor layer. Relatively weak backscatter returns from the choroid and appears green on the tomogram. The intermediate layers, between the highly reflective NFL and RPE, exhibit moderate backscatter and are represented on the false color scale as yellow-green.

NONEXUDATIVE AGE-RELATED MACULAR DEGENERATION (DRUSEN AND GEOGRAPHIC ATROPHY)

Nonexudative AMD can cause patterns of hyperfluorescence on fluorescein angiography that must be distinguished from exudative or neovascular lesions. Both drusen and geographic atrophy produce characteristic features. These lesions may also be imaged by OCT.

Drusen appear on angiography as punctate areas of hyperfluorescence. Staining occurs in the early phase and generally diminishes in the later phases, although larger drusen may retain fluorescein and exhibit continued late hyperfluorescence. On OCT, soft drusen cause a modulation in the highly reflective posterior boundary of the retina consistent with the

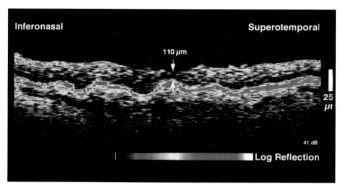

Figure 3-7. OCT of drusen.

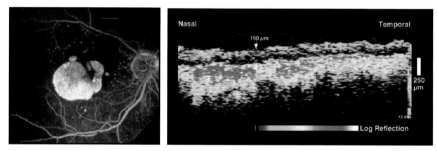

Figure 3-8. Fluorescein angiogram and OCT of geographic atrophy.

accumulation of material within the RPE (Figure 3-7). The small elevations of the RPE can appear similar to RPE detachments just as fluorescein angiography of large drusen can resemble pooling under RPE detachments.

Geographic atrophy occurs as patches of attenuated RPE in the macula. On fluorescein angiography, there is transmission of normal choroidal fluorescein as a window defect. The timing of hyperfluorescence coincides with filling of the choriocapillaris and diminishes as the choroid empties. In contrast to CNV, the borders of hyperfluorescence remain fixed at the boundaries of RPE atrophy. OCT shows thinning of the overlying retina. The hypopigmented RPE allows deeper penetration of the incident light into the choroid. The choroidal layer will have higher than normal backscatter due to a decrease in signal absorption from the atrophic retina and RPE (Figure 3-8).

EXUDATIVE AGE-RELATED MACULAR DEGENERATION

Classic Choroidal Neovascularization

Classic CNV was defined by the MPS using fluorescein angiographic criteria. A classic lesion exhibits bright, uniform early hyperfluorescence, normally within the first 30 seconds. The lesion leaks in the late phase, typically with obscuration of the boundaries of CNV (Figure 3-9). Blockage by hemorrhage, lipid, or pigment may obscure the boundaries of classic CNV (Figure 3-10).[6]

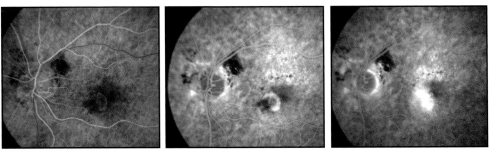

Figure 3-9. Fluorescein angiography of classic CNV.

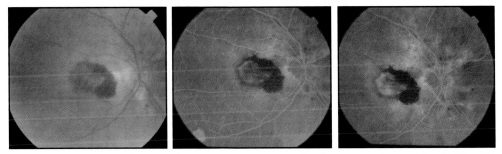

Figure 3-10. Color photo and fluorescein angiography demonstrating classic CNV with boundaries obscured by blocking hemorrhage.

Occult Choroidal Neovascularization

Occult CNV was also defined by the MPS using fluorescein angiographic criteria. The lesions may manifest as a fibrovascular PED or late leakage of undetermined source.

A fibrovascular PED shows an irregular elevation of the RPE on stereoscopic angiography. Stippled hyperfluorescence is evident within 1 to 2 minutes after fluorescein injection. There is persistence of staining or leakage in the late phases of the angiogram (Figure 3-11).

Late leakage from an undetermined source represents fluorescein leakage at the level of the RPE in the late phase of the angiogram without a discernable corresponding source of leakage in the early phase. The appearance is often described as speckled.

Optical Coherence Tomography of Choroidal Neovascularization

The presentation of CNV on OCT typically falls into one of three categories but may show variability. Neovascular complexes that are angiographically well-defined typically present as fusiform enlargement of the RPE/choriocapillaris reflective band with discrete borders (Figure 3-12). Occasionally, the membrane may be imaged in the subretinal space (Figure 3-13). Neovascular complexes that are poorly defined angiographically and fall into the category of occult fibrovascular PEDs display a well-defined elevation of the RPE reflective band with a mildly backscattering region below, corresponding to fibrous proliferation (Figure 3-14). No shadowing of the choroidal reflection is present. Many choroidal neovascular complexes display enhanced choroidal reflection without a discrete membrane. This may be due to increased optical penetration secondary to RPE changes.[1]

Figure 3-11. Fluorescein angiography of occult fibrovascular PED.

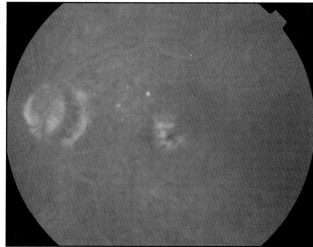

Figure 3-12. Fluorescein angiography and OCT of classic CNV demonstrating fusiform hyper-reflective complex beneath the neurosensory retina. The optically clear spaces adjacent to the CNV are collections of subretinal fluid.

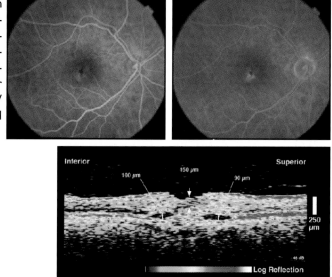

The presence of intraretinal fluid may be represented as retinal thickening or as the accumulation of fluid in well-defined spaces. Intraretinal fluid in localized cysts (cystoid macular edema) appears as areas of discrete decreases in backscatter within the intermediate retinal layers (Figure 3-15), while diffuse edema will show an increase in thickness without definite spaces (Figure 3-16). Neurosensory detachments from the accumulation of subretinal fluid appear in cross-section as elevations of the neurosensory retina above an optically clear space (Figure 3-17). The fluid space has well-defined boundaries at the fluid-retinal and fluid-RPE interfaces. In contrast to RPE detachments, the highly reflective RPE is imaged at the posterior border of the detachment.

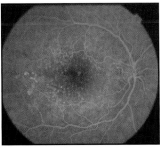
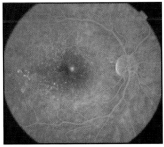

Figure 3-13. Small neovascular complex on fluorescein angiography imaged in the subretinal space by OCT. The highly reflective band anterior to the RPE/choriocapillaris layer represents the CNV.

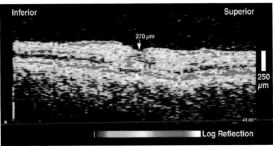

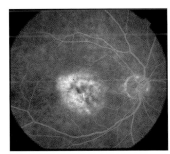
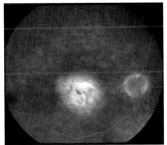

Figure 3-14. Fluorescein angiography and OCT of occult fibrovascular PED.

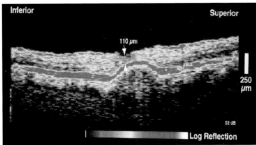

SEROUS AND HEMORRHAGIC RETINAL PIGMENT EPITHELIAL DETACHMENTS

A serous detachment of the RPE is represented as a uniform elevation of the RPE that is often circular. On fluorescein angiography, there is uniform pooling within the PED starting in the early phase and progressing through the late phase. The borders remain confined by the limits of the RPE detachment. Bright hyperfluorescence persists throughout the angiogram (Figure 3-18). A hemorrhagic PED shows blocked fluorescence due to the presence of opaque blood between the RPE and underlying choriocapillaris.

Figure 3-15. Fluorescein angiography and OCT demonstrating cystoid macular edema associated with classic CNV.

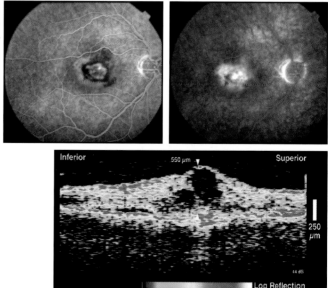

Figure 3-16. Fluorescein angiography and OCT demonstrating diffuse intraretinal edema associated with classic CNV.

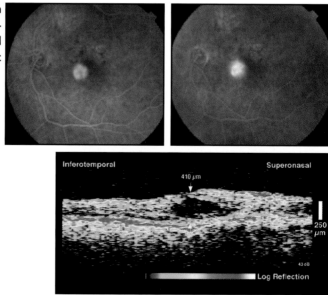

It is possible to distinguish between serous and hemorrhagic RPE detachments based on OCT images. Serous PEDs appear as dome-shaped elevations of the RPE with an elevated reflective band corresponding to the RPE. The intervening nonreflective layer is fluid in the sub-RPE space. The margins are sharp, and there typically is shadowing of the reflections returning from the deeper choroid. This may be due to increased reflectivity and attenuation of the light through the decompensated RPE. Hemorrhagic PEDs have a similar appearance. However, images of hemorrhagic detachments tend to show a band of high backscatter under the RPE band at the apex of the detachment (Figure 3-19). This corresponds to

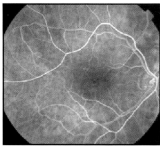
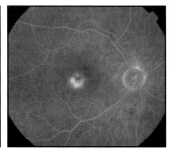

Figure 3-17. Fluorescein angiography and OCT demonstrating subretinal fluid associated with classic CNV.

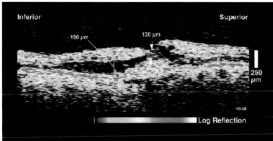

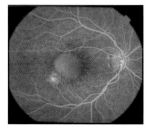
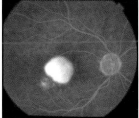

Figure 3-18. Fluorescein angiography and OCT demonstrating serous PED. Compared to a hemorrhagic PED on OCT, serous PEDs have an optically empty cavity under the RPE with a reflective choroidal layer.

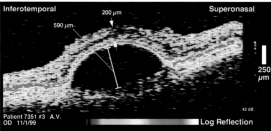

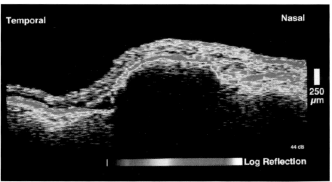

Figure 3-19. OCT of hemorrhagic PED. Note shadowing of the posterior signal by anterior hemorrhage under the RPE/choriocapillaris band.

Figure 3-20. Fluorescein angiography demonstrating late staining of a chronic, predominantly fibrotic lesion.

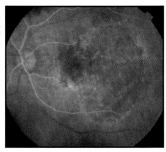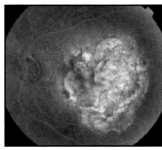

the accumulated blood, decreasing light penetration, and attenuating choroidal reflection. Hemorrhagic PEDs and subretinal hemorrhages are sometimes difficult to distinguish on OCT because blood and the detached RPE have similar reflectivity.

SUBRETINAL FIBROSIS/DISCIFORM SCARRING

The end-stage of regressed CNV results in subretinal fibrosis or disciform scarring. This consists of white, fibrous tissue between the retina and RPE or below the RPE. Scars may show blocked fluorescence and/or staining on fluorescein angiography. This tissue is highly reflective on OCT and frequently shows overlying retinal atrophy (Figure 3-20).

SUMMARY

A strong understanding of fluorescein angiography patterns is necessary for effective use of PDT in patients with CNV secondary to AMD. Proper interpretation will allow the treatment of lesions that demonstrate a statistically significant benefit from PDT in the TAP Study. Similarly, lesions may be excluded that do not respond to treatment, including drusen, geographic atrophy, serous/hemorrhagic PEDs, disciform scars, and lesions. Further studies may expand the indications to a broader spectrum of lesions in the future.

OCT is a noninvasive imaging modality capable of providing accurate, reproducible images of the posterior segment. The retinal and RPE changes in AMD have a characteristic appearance on OCT. OCT is useful in detecting small changes in retinal thickness, subretinal and sub-RPE fluid, and CNV. It accurately localizes these processes and may provide an objective measurement. This is particularly useful in monitoring the response to PDT in concert with conventional fluorescein and indocyanine green angiography.

REFERENCES

1. Puliafito CA, Hee MR, Schuman JS, et al. *Optical Coherence Tomography of Ocular Diseases.* Thorofare, NJ: SLACK Incorporated; 1996.

2. Hee MR, Puliafito CA, Duker JS, et al. Topography of diabetic macular edema with optical coherence tomography. *Ophthalmology.* 1998;105:360-370.

3. Puliafito CA, Hee MR, Lin CP, et al. Imaging of macular diseases with optical coherence tomography. *Ophthalmology.* 1995;102:217-229.

4. Hee MR, Puliafito CA, Wong C, et al. Optical coherence tomography macular holes. *Ophthalmology.* 1995;102:748-756.

5. Hee MR, Baumal C, Puliafito CA, et al. Optical coherence tomography of age-related macular degeneration and choroidal neovascularization. *Ophthalmology*. 1996;103:1260-1270.

6. Macular Photocoagulation Study Group. Subfoveal neovascular lesions in age-related macular degeneration: guidelines for evaluation and treatment in the macular photocoagulation study. *Arch Ophthalmol*. 1991;109:1242-1257.

7. Treatment of Age-Related Macular Degeneration with Photodynamic Therapy Study Group. Photodynamic therapy of subfoveal choroidal neovascularization in age-related macular degeneration with verteporfin: two-year results of two randomized clinical trials—TAP Report #2. *Arch Ophthalmol*. 2001;119:198-207.

CHAPTER FOUR

TREATMENT OF SUBFOVEAL CHOROIDAL NEOVASCULARIZATION SECONDARY TO AGE-RELATED MACULAR DEGENERATION

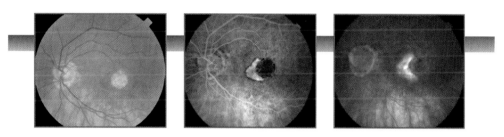

CHAPTER SECTIONS

MACULAR PHOTOCOAGULATION STUDY

Given the poor visual outcomes with untreated subfoveal choroidal neovascularization (CNV) from age-related macular degeneration (AMD), research has focused on treatment (Table 4-1). In 1986, the Macular Photocoagulation Study Group (MPS) concurrently began two randomized trials evaluating the efficacy of laser photocoagulation of CNV under the geometric center of the foveal avascular zone (FAZ). The two trials, independently published in 1991, evaluated the treatment of primary subfoveal CNV secondary to AMD and subfoveal CNV originating from the edge of a laser photocoagulation scar.[1,2] The results of these trials demonstrated a statistically significant, albeit modest, improvement over the natural course of disease when subfoveal CNV meeting the MPS eligibility criteria was treated with photocoagulation. As a disclaimer, the MPS authors advised that laser treatment should commence as long as both the ophthalmologist and patient were prepared for an immediate decline in visual acuity.[3,4]

In both trials, the patients were randomly assigned to receive either photocoagulation treatment or observation (Table 4-2). The goal of each trial was to photocoagulate the entire CNV, thus requiring the lesion to be well-demarcated with a visible edge. A component of classic CNV was required for treatment in all cases. Eyes with occult CNV without evidence of classic CNV were ineligible even if the entire lesion had well-demarcated boundaries. Eligible eyes required some area of uninvolved retina within 1500 microns of the center of the FAZ that would remain untreated. In primary subfoveal CNV, the lesion could not exceed 3.5 standard disc areas (1 disc area, 1.77 mm^2). In eyes with recurrent subfoveal CNV, the previous treatment scar and neovascular lesion could not exceed 6 disc areas (10.6 mm^2). Lesion components such as subretinal hemorrhage, serous detachment of the retinal pigment epithelium (RPE), and elevated blocked hypofluorescence could be present, but the total area occupied by the CNV had to be proportionally greater than the area occupied by the lesion components (Figure 4-1). During treatment, all components of the lesion were photocoagulated, including an area extending 100 microns beyond the peripheral boundary of all lesion components except blood. Thick blood only required laser treatment up to the edge of uninvolved retina. When treating at the junction of CNV and laser scar in recurrent subfoveal lesions, photocoagulation was extended 300 microns into the adjacent laser scar. When present in the recurrent lesions, feeder vessels were treated 100 microns beyond the lateral border of the vessels and 300 microns radially beyond the origin. The parameters for photocoagulation required a 200- to 500-micron spot with a 0.2- to 0.5-second duration to create a border 100 microns beyond the lesion except for thick blood as described above. The body of the lesion was then treated with burns of the same spot size, but with the duration increased to 0.5- to 1.0-second. The goal of photocoagulation was to create a uniformly white lesion representing a full-thickness retinal burn.[3]

In the randomized clinical trial evaluating the treatment of primary subfoveal CNV secondary to AMD with no treatment, 189 eyes were treated with laser photocoagulation as described above. A statistically significant difference in visual acuity in the treatment group was not observed until the 24-month evaluation. At 3 months, 184 eyes that received laser were examined with a mean visual acuity of 20/320 compared with 20/200 in the untreated group. At 24 months, the mean visual acuity in the 114 treated eyes remained at 20/320 while the untreated eyes declined to 20/400. Treated eyes experienced an immediate 3-line decrease in visual acuity that was not observed in the control group. However, the visual loss stabilized after month 3. At 24 months, treated eyes declined an average of 3 lines in visual acuity from baseline compared with 4.4 lines in the no-treatment group.[1]

TABLE 4-1

CHANGE IN VISUAL ACUITY FROM INITIAL VISIT COMPARING TREATMENT AND CONTROL GROUPS IN VARIOUS STUDIES

MPS (Primary Subfoveal CNV)[1]	Month	Mean Lines Lost	Mean Visual Acuity
Treatment group	3	3.0	20/320
	24	3.0	20/320
Control group	3	1.9	20/200
	24	4.4	20/400
MPS (Recurrent Subfoveal CNV)[2]			
Treatment group	3	2.4	20/250
	24	2.7	20/250
Control group	3	1.7	20/200
	24	3.4	20/320
RAD Study[5]			
Treatment group	12	3.5	
Control group	12	3.7	
Submacular Surgery Trial[6]			
Surgery group	24	2.0	20/200
Laser group	24	0	20/200

MPS = Macular Photocoagulation Study
RAD = Radiation for Age-Related Macular Degeneration

TABLE 4-2

OVERVIEW OF MPS ELIGIBILITY CRITERIA AND TREATMENT PARAMETERS FOR PRIMARY AND RECURRENT SUBFOVEAL CNV[1-3]

1. Primarily classic CNV <3.5 MPS disc areas; <6 disc areas in recurrent subfoveal CNV (includes the CNV, treatment scar, and feeder vessels).
2. Well-demarcated lesion borders.
3. Blood, hypofluorescent rim, and lipid-blocking fluorescence may be present as long as the CNV occupies a greater proportion of the lesion.
4. Snellen equivalent visual acuity of 20/40 to 20/320 on a Bailey-Lovie visual acuity chart.
5. Treatment should be extended 100 microns beyond the perimeter of the lesion, 300 microns into the adjacent laser scar, to the edge of hemorrhage.
6. Feeder vessels are treated 100 microns beyond the edge and 300 microns beyond the base of the vessel.
7. Laser burns to create full-thickness retinal whitening.
   a. 200- to 500-micron spot with 0.2- to 0.5-second duration of argon green or krypton red.

Figure 4-1. Depiction of CNV with various lesion components.

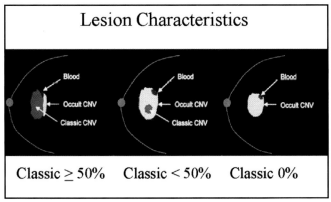

Figure 4-2. A 46-year-old male with diffuse macular drusen complained of metamorphopsia (A). Fluorescein angiography demonstrated a punctate area of hyperfluorescence in mid (B) and late frames (C). Triamcinolone acetonide 4 mg was injected into the vitreous cavity. Symptoms subsided and fluorescein angiography 1 month after intravitreal steroids demonstrated resolution of the

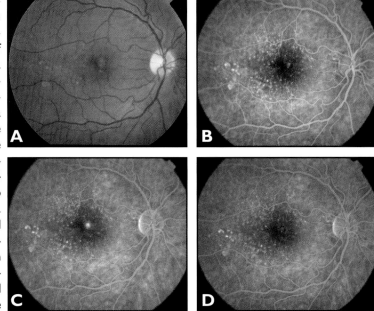

CNV (D). The patient remained asymptomatic for 1 year when metamorphopsia returned with recurrent CNV on angiography (E). The patient was reinjected with triamcinolone acetonide 4 mg.

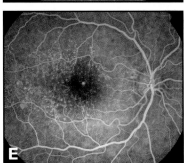

Similar results were found in the randomized clinical trial evaluating photocoagulation of recurrent subfoveal CNV originating from prior laser scar for the treatment of extrafoveal or juxtafoveal CNV from AMD, ocular histoplasmosis, or idiopathic CNV.[2] An immediate decrease of 3 lines of visual acuity occurred after treatment, followed by stabilization. The control group lost 1.7 lines at 3 months followed by a mean decline of 3.4 lines at 24 months. The mean visual acuity in the treatment group was 20/250 at the 3-month visit and remained at this level at the 24-month examination. The average visual acuity of the control group was 20/200 at 3 months declining to 20/320 at 24 months. These visual acuity results between the two groups were not statistically significant.

In summary, treated eyes that met MPS criteria 2 years after enrollment had marginally better visual acuity than untreated eyes. For the initial 3 months, eyes that received photocoagulation experienced a rapid decline in visual acuity followed by stabilization. Treated eyes were less likely to experience severe visual loss (decrease of 6 or more lines) than untreated eyes by 24 months. Regardless of the results, treating ophthalmologists were urged to discuss with their patients the risk of experiencing immediate visual loss, as laser photocoagulation irreversibly destroys the overlying neurosensory retina.

RADIATION THERAPY FOR AGE-RELATED MACULAR DEGENERATION STUDY

The Radiation Therapy for Age-Related Macular Degeneration (RAD) Study Group evaluated the efficacy of external beam radiation therapy of CNV secondary to AMD in a prospective, randomized, double-blinded trial.[5] This represents the first study of radiation to utilize a control group with sham treatment. Eligible patients had subfoveal classic or occult CNV with a lesion size of 6 disc areas or less, visual acuity of 20/320 or better, visual symptoms of 6 months or less, and absence of foveal hemorrhage. One hundred one patients were randomized to receive eight fractions of 2 Gy external beam irradiation, while 104 patients received eight fractions of a sham treatment.

One year after randomization, 183 patients (89.3%) were available for follow-up examinations. No adverse effects from the radiation therapy were noted during the 12 months of follow-up including radiation retinopathy or optic neuropathy. Of the 88 patients receiving radiation treatment examined at 1 year, the mean decrease in visual acuity was 3.5 lines compared with a 3.7-line drop experienced by the 95 patients in the control group. No statistically significant difference existed whether classic or occult CNV was present either in the treatment or control group. Three or more lines of visual acuity were lost in 51.1% of the treated and 52.6% of the controls at 1 year. In general, external beam radiation administered at a dose of 16 Gy applied in eight fractions of 2 Gy provided no statistically significant benefit for the treatment of subfoveal classic or occult CNV secondary to AMD.

The authors did not rule out that an alternate dose of radiation may improve visual outcome as they speculated that the overall dose of radiation used in the trial might have been too small to close the CNV. However, higher doses of radiation to the eye impart a greater risk of adverse events. In addition, the treatment group in the masked, randomized trial presented by the RAD Study Group did not even demonstrate a trend toward an improved functional outcome.[5] The use of radiation has therefore lost favor for the treatment of CNV secondary to AMD.

SUBMACULAR SURGERY TRIAL

Submacular surgery involves the creation of a retinotomy to gain access to the subretinal space during pars plana vitrectomy. Surgical removal of CNV with associated scar and blood has gained recent popularity as an alternative to foveal laser treatment. The theoretical advantage is that some of the macular photoreceptors will be preserved despite the loss of RPE.[6] Whereas laser treatment of CNV requires well-demarcated boundaries, lesions with poorly demarcated borders are amenable to surgical excision, expanding the population that may be treated. The Submacular Surgery Trial (SST) Pilot Study represents the first study to evaluate the efficacy of submacular surgery compared with laser photocoagulation for the treatment of subfoveal CNV.

Patients were eligible if they had a recurrent subfoveal CNV originating from the edge of a prior laser scar from previous photocoagulation of extrafoveal or juxtafoveal CNV secondary to AMD. The total lesion size could not exceed 9 MPS disc areas, which included the prior laser scar, recurrent CNV, and any lesion components that block fluorescence. While classic CNV was required, the subfoveal portion of the lesion could be occult or classic. Entry into the trial required a visual acuity ranging from 20/64 to 20/800. The goal of the submacular surgery was to remove the entire choroidal neovascular lesion including occult and classic CNV, subretinal blood, and scar.

Of the 70 patients enrolled in the SST, 36 were randomized to laser and 34 to submacular surgery when the study was closed in 1997. The mean baseline visual acuity at enrollment was 20/160 in both groups. The median visual acuity in both treatment arms remained 20/200 to 20/250 throughout the 24-month follow-up period with 89% of patients in the laser group and 85% in the surgical group returning for follow-up at 2 years. At the 24-month exam, 26% of the laser treated eyes and 14% of the surgically treated eyes improved by 2 or more lines of visual acuity. Of all patients, the surgical group on average lost 2 lines of visual acuity, while the laser group remained stable.

The SST concluded that surgical removal of recurrent subfoveal CNV provided no benefit over laser photocoagulation. Given that laser photocoagulation has been proven beneficial by the MPS and that submacular surgery failed to provide a visual benefit in any subgroup, the Data and Safety Monitoring Committee halted further recruitment of patients for the trial. The investigators recommended that laser photocoagulation be the first line of treatment for recurrent subfoveal CNV secondary to AMD.[6]

TRANSPUPILLARY THERMOTHERAPY

Transpupillary thermotherapy (TTT) has emerged as a recent advancement for the treatment of occult subfoveal CNV in patients with AMD. TTT is administered through a slit lamp-mounted delivery system attached to a modified infrared diode laser at 810 nm (Iris Medical Instruments, Mountain View, Calif). The beam has an adjustable width of 1.2 mm, 2.0 mm, and 3.0 mm and is transmitted to the retina via a diode-coated contact lens. The beam width may be further enlarged through contact lens magnification. Treatment is initiated when the entire spot envelopes the visible retinal lesion. The typical power settings range between 360 and 1000 mW based on the diameter of the spot size, fundus pigmentation, choroidal blood flow, and media clarity.[7]

TTT treats occult CNV in a subthreshold manner with long exposure and large retinal spot sizes. At 810 nm, the energy transmitted to the eye penetrates to the choroid and RPE while minimizing absorption in the neurosensory retina. The choroidal vasculature further acts to dissipate generated heat. In contrast to threshold treatment from conventional short-pulsed photocoagulation where an estimated rise in retinal temperature of 42°C occurs, the estimated retinal temperature elevation with TTT at standard settings (800 mW, 60 seconds, 3.0 mm spot size) is approximately 10°C.[7] Through this delivery of thermal energy to the choroid, the mechanism of treatment of CNV by TTT may occur through vascular thrombosis, apoptosis, or the thermal inhibition of angiogenesis.[7]

Initially used in the treatment of choroidal melanomas,[8,9] a recent pilot study of 16 eyes in 15 patients with occult subfoveal CNV treated with TTT demonstrated the effectiveness of this form of treatment in stabilizing visual acuity.[10] With a mean follow-up of 12 months, three of 16 eyes (19%) improved by 2 or more lines of Snellen visual acuity. Nine eyes (56%) had no change in visual acuity, and four eyes (25%) declined by 2 or more lines. Fifteen of the 16 eyes treated with TTT demonstrated improvement in the amount of exudation. Diminished exudation was also present in three of four eyes that experienced a decline in visual acuity.

Miller-Rivero and Kaplan[11] treated 30 eyes with TTT of which 22 were predominantly occult and eight were predominantly classic. Pretreatment visual acuity ranged from 20/40 to counting fingers. Eight eyes (26.7%) improved 2 lines or more, 13 eyes (43.3%) remained within 1 line of pretreatment visual acuity, and nine eyes (30.0%) declined 2 or more lines. Twenty-six eyes demonstrated a decrease in exudation after treatment, and seven eyes were retreated.[11]

Newsome and associates[12] further evaluated the efficacy of TTT for the treatment of both classic and occult CNV. In a nonrandomized fashion, 44 eyes of 42 patients with symptomatic visual loss and angiographic evidence of CNV secondary to AMD were enrolled for treatment. Twelve of the lesions were predominantly classic and 32 predominantly occult. The study population also included 11 eyes with serous pigment epithelial detachments. In the predominantly occult group, 78% of the lesions were closed with an average of 0.66 Snellen lines lost over 7.2 months of follow-up. Predominantly classic lesions were closed in 75% of eyes with an average of 0.75 Snellen lines lost. Stabilization or improvement in visual acuity occurred in 71% of eyes with occult lesions and 67% of eyes with classic lesions.

While the results are promising for stabilizing vision, TTT remains an unproven technique for the treatment of occult subfoveal CNV. TTT is currently being investigated in a randomized, double-blind, multicenter trial.

ANTI-ANGIOGENIC AGENTS

Given the damage to photoreceptors from laser photocoagulation, alternative therapies have focused on anti-angiogenic agents to inhibit vascular endothelial proliferation. The Pharmacologic Therapy for Macular Degeneration Study Group evaluated interferon alpha-2a for the treatment of CNV from AMD.[13] Eligible lesions included classic and occult CNV that were either primary or recurrent lesions. The interferon was administered subcutaneously in three different strengths and compared to placebo. At 1 year, 38% of placebo-treated patients and 50% of interferon alpha-2a treatment patients lost 3 or more lines of vision. No visual benefit from interferon was seen in any subgroup analysis. Signs of interferon-associated retinopathy consisting of retinal hemorrhages and cotton wool spots were noted with increasing frequency in a dose-dependent fashion. The authors concluded that interferon alpha-2a provided no benefit for the treatment of CNV secondary to AMD.[13]

Triamcinolone acetonide is a corticosteroid with anti-inflammatory properties initiated by the inhibition of arachidonic acid formation. In addition, triamcinolone has intrinsic anti-angiogenic properties. Danis et al[14] evaluated the efficacy of a 4.0 mg dose of triamcinolone acetonide injected into the vitreous cavity for the treatment of subfoveal classic or occult CNV from AMD. Sixteen patients with CNV and visual acuity ranging from 20/40 to 20/400 received intravitreal triamcinolone acetonide and were compared to 11 untreated eyes for 6 months. At 6 months, the mean visual acuity had improved 0.04 logMAR units in the treated eyes compared with a decline of 0.39 units in the control eyes. This decline in visual acuity measured at both 3 and 6 months in the untreated control group was statistically significant. Despite a nonstatistically significant improvement in visual acuity in the treatment group, the fluorescein angiogram in some of the treatment patients exhibited increased exudation. This may indicate that intravitreous-injected corticosteroids may have only a modest effect on the natural history of subfoveal CNV.[14] Side effects encountered included cataract formation and intraocular pressure (IOP) elevation. Elevated IOP was identified in 25% of patients and successfully controlled with ocular hypotensive agents.

Intravitreal triamcinolone acetonide appears to be a promising treatment for CNV as photoreceptor damage is avoided by the treatment. Further evaluation in a multicenter, blinded, placebo-controlled trial with longer follow-up is needed to accurately assess the efficacy of this treatment.

MACULAR TRANSLOCATION

Macular translocation is a procedure that surgically detaches the fovea occupied by CNV and scar, relocating it to an extrafoveal location where it may be treated with laser photocoagulation or photodynamic therapy. Lewis and associates[15] evaluated 10 eyes of 10 patients older than 60 years of age with classic and occult subfoveal CNV from AMD and visual acuity between 20/50 and 20/800. The CNV was either primary or recurrent, involved the geometric center of the FAZ, and measured 6 MPS disc areas or less. Translocation of the fovea occurred through scleral imbrication, pars plana vitrectomy, intentional retinal detachment for 180 to 240 degrees by infusing balanced salt solution into the subretinal space through multiple retinotomies, and a partial air-fluid exchange without drainage of the subretinal fluid. The patient was maintained in an upright position postoperatively to allow inferior displacement of the fovea. Lesions successfully translocated to an extrafoveal location were photocoagulated on postoperative day 1.[15]

All 10 eyes exhibited reattachment of the retina 6 months after the initial surgery. The fovea was displaced an average of 1286 microns from its original position. Visual acuity improved in four eyes and declined in six eyes. The average preoperative visual acuity measured 20/111 with a postoperative visual acuity of 20/160. Nine of 10 eyes were 20/250 or better, but no eye achieved a final visual acuity better than 20/80. Complications with the procedure included retinal detachment, retinal folds through the fovea, image distortion or tilting, and rhegmatogenous retinal detachment.

The advantage of macular translocation is that it can treat both classic and occult CNV with poorly defined margins. Due to the unpredictability of the procedure and potential surgical complications, Lewis et al concluded that further refinement of the surgical technique was required.[15]

References

1. Macular Photocoagulation Study Group. Laser photocoagulation of subfoveal neovascular lesions in age-related macular degeneration: results of a randomized clinical trial. *Arch Ophthalmol.* 1991;109:1220-1231.

2. Macular Photocoagulation Study Group. Laser photocoagulation of subfoveal recurrent neovascular lesions in age-related macular degeneration: results of a randomized clinical trial. *Arch Ophthalmol.* 1991;109:1232-1241.

3. Macular Photocoagulation Study Group. Subfoveal neovascular lesions in age-related macular degeneration: guidelines for evaluation and treatment in the macular photocoagulation study. *Arch Ophthalmol.* 1991;109:1242-1257.

4. Schachat AP. Management of subfoveal choroidal neovascularization (editorial). *Arch Ophthalmol.* 1991;109:1217-1218.

5. The Radiation Therapy for Age-Related Macular Degeneration (RAD) Study Group. A prospective, randomized, double-masked trial on radiation therapy for neovascular age-related macular degeneration (RAD Study). *Ophthalmology.* 1999;106:2239-2247.

6. Submacular Surgery Trials Pilot Study Investigators. Submacular surgery trials randomized pilot trial of laser photocoagulation versus surgery for recurrent choroidal neovascularization secondary to age-related macular degeneration: I. Ophthalmic outcomes: submacular surgery trials pilot study report number 1. *Am J Ophthalmol.* 2000;130:387-407.

7. Mainster MA, Reichel E. Transpupillary thermotherapy for age-related macular degeneration: long-pulse photocoagulation, apoptosis, and heat shock proteins. *Ophthalmic Surg Lasers.* 2000;31:359-373.

8. Shields CL, Shields JA, DePotter P, Kheterpal S. Transpupillary thermotherapy in the management of choroidal melanoma. *Ophthalmology.* 1996;103:1642-1650.

9. Shields CL, Shields JA, Cater J, et al. Transpupillary thermotherapy for choroidal melanoma. Tumor control and visual results in 100 consecutive cases. *Ophthalmology.* 1998;105:581-590.

10. Reichel E, Berrocal AM, Ip M, et al. Transpupillary thermotherapy of occult subfoveal choroidal neovascularization in patients with age-related macular degeneration. *Ophthalmology.* 1999;106:1908-1914.

11. Miller-Rivero NE, Kaplan HJ. Transpupillary thermotherapy in the treatment of occult choroidal neovascularization. *Invest Ophthalmol Vis Sci.* 2000;41:S179.

12. Newsome RSB, McAlister JC, Saeed M, McHugh JDA. Transpupillary thermotherapy (TTT) for the treatment of choroidal neovascularisation. *Br J Ophthalmol.* 2001;85:173-178.

13. Pharmacologic Therapy for Macular Degeneration Study Group. Interferon alpha-2a is ineffective for patients with choroidal neovascularization secondary to age-related macular degeneration: results of a prospective randomized placebo controlled clinical trial. *Arch Ophthalmol.* 1997;115:865-872.

14. Danis RP, Ciulla TA, Pratt LM, Anliker W. Intravitreal triamcinolone acetonide in exudative age-related macular degeneration. *Retina.* 2000;20:244-250.

15. Lewis H, Kaiser P, Lewis S, Estafanous M. Macular translocation for subfoveal choroidal neovascularization in age-related macular degeneration: a prospective study. *Am J Ophthalmol.* 1999;128:135-146.

CHAPTER FIVE

PHOTOSENSITIZING AGENTS

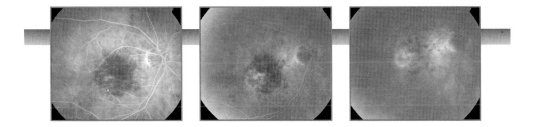

CHAPTER SECTIONS

❖ Benzoporphyrin Derivative Monoacid (Verteporfin)

❖ Tin Ethyl Etiopurpurin (SnET2)

❖ Lutetium Texaphyrin

❖ ATX-S10(Na)

❖ Chloroaluminum Sulfonated Phthalocyanine (CASPc)

❖ Mono-L-Aspartyl Chlorin e6 (NPe6)

❖ Conclusion

Treatment of choroidal neovascularization (CNV) with thermal laser photocoagulation has been limited by narrow eligibility requirements, high recurrence rates, and the potential complication of permanent scotomata from heat-induced damage to the overlying retinal pigment epithelium (RPE) and neurosensory retina.[1] This is especially problematic in patients with subfoveal CNV who experience immediate and irreversible central visual loss after photocoagulation.[2,3] Photodynamic therapy (PDT) has evolved to treat CNV without the complications of standard laser photocoagulation. Originally developed as an experimental treatment of solid tumors, PDT is employed to selectively occlude CNV while minimizing the degree of injury to the surrounding neurosensory retina.[4-6]

The basic mechanism of PDT is light activation of a photosensitizing agent based on its absorption profile. Treatment requires systemic intravenous administration of a sensitizing dye, which selectively distributes in CNV. Photosensitizers have a high affinity for proliferating neovascular tissue[7] and plasma proteins, especially low density lipoproteins (LDL). The endothelium of neovascular tissue exhibits increased LDL receptors compared to the surrounding normal vascular endothelium. The LDL-bound photosensitizer complex is preferentially transported across the vascular endothelium and localized in the CNV.[8-10]

Activation of the photochemical is initiated by laser delivery of wavelength-specific, nonthermal light to the CNV.[11-13] After light activation, the photosensitizer is converted either to an excited state that decays back to the ground state with fluorescence or to a longer lived, lower energy triplet state. This more stable triplet state may decay with phosphorescence or interact directly with oxygen in either a Type I or Type II reaction.[11,14,15] Type I reactions involve the production of hydroxyl radicals, peroxides, and superoxides. Type II reactions involve a direct interaction with oxygen to produce singlet oxygen. Type II reactions are believed to play a primary role in PDT-mediated phototoxicity.[11,14-16] Singlet oxygen possesses a reactive distance of only 0.1 micron, restricting cytotoxicity to the immediate vicinity of the photosensitized drug.[17] A local inflammatory response is initiated with the production of prostaglandin E2, interleukin-2, interleukin-1β, and tumor necrosis factor-α.[18,19] Occlusion of the vascular bed occurs with damage to the vascular endothelial cells, platelet adhesion and aggregation, and subsequent thrombus formation.[16]

The clinical effectiveness of a photosensitizer is closely linked to its pharmacokinetic and pharmacodynamic properties. The ideal photosensitizer should have a long absorption wavelength for improved tissue penetration, remain water-soluble, be minimally toxic, localize to abnormal vascular tissue, and be rapidly eliminated from the body. This chapter describes the current photosensitizing agents involved in the clinical and experimental treatment of CNV (Table 5-1).

BENZOPORPHYRIN DERIVATIVE MONOACID (VERTEPORFIN)

Benzoporphyrin derivative monoacid (BPD), a second-generation photosensitizer approved for use by the US Food and Drug Administration for the treatment of subfoveal CNV due to age-related macular degeneration (AMD), is marketed under the trade name Visudyne (Novartis Ophthalmics, Duluth, Ga). It has peak absorption at 689 nm.[20] BPD is administered intravenously and preferentially associates with lipoproteins upon mixture with human plasma. Prebinding of BPD to LDL leads to delayed clearance and enhanced delivery to target tissues as cellular uptake is mediated almost entirely by LDL receptors.[21-24] This BPD-LDL complex is viewed as the standard mode of delivery to neovascular tissue.

BPD is cleared from the blood rapidly during the first 24 hours post-injection. Hepatic metabolism with biliary excretion is the main route of elimination, with 60% of the inject-

TABLE 5-1

PHOTOSENSITIZING AGENTS

Photosensitizer	Wavelength (nm)
Verteporfin	689
SnET2	664
Lutetium texaphyrin	732
ATX-S10(Na)	670
CASPc	675
NPe6	664

ed dose cleared through the feces during the first 24 hours. The clearance rate from the liver is biphasic.[23,25] The first phase of rapid clearance has a decay rate of 0.15 min[-1] and a $t_{1/2}$ of less than 20 minutes. The second phase is slower and has a decay rate of 0.0013 min[-1] and a $t_{1/2}$ of 530 minutes.[23]

Biodistribution studies demonstrate high BPD levels in the liver, spleen, gall bladder, and kidneys.[25] In the eye, BPD has the highest concentrations in vascular structures such as the iris, ciliary body, and choroid, with avascular structures such as the sclera, cornea, lens, and vitreous showing minimal accumulation. The RPE, with a high concentration of LDL receptors, rapidly accumulates BPD.[23] Based on angiographic studies in monkeys with indocyanine green and fluorescein,[26] BPD reaches the choroidal vessels 5 to 7 seconds after injection and persists for up to 60 minutes. BPD is detectable in the retinal vasculature 10 to 15 seconds after injection. Clearance from the retina begins at 15 minutes and is complete by 30 minutes after an intravenous bolus injection. BPD is present in CNV 10 seconds after injection, persisting for a maximum of 60 minutes.

BPD is well-tolerated systemically with few side effects. Twelve percent of patients in the Treatment of Age-Related Macular Degeneration with Photodynamic Therapy (TAP) Study experienced photosensitivity reactions.[6] Other adverse effects included visual disturbances and injection site events such as edema and extravasation. Less common adverse events include vitreous hemorrhage, retinal capillary nonperfusion, infusion-related back pain, and allergic reactions. Most importantly, BPD does not cause any significant skin photosensitivity past 24 hours post-injection.[25]

TIN ETHYL ETIOPURPURIN (SNET2)

Tin ethyl etiopurpurin (SnET2) is a second-generation, highly hydrophobic photosensitizer with an absorption peak at 664 nm.[27] SnET2 is administered intravenously as an isotonic, iso-osmotic lipid emulsion with an affinity for the high-density lipoprotein (HDL) partitions of plasma.[28,29]

PDT with SnET2 in animal models suggests selective targeting of the choriocapillaris. Histological examination of rabbit eyes irradiated with light at a fluence of 20 J/cm[2] confirmed choriocapillaris closure, with reperfusion occurring by day 28.[29] The optimal time for occlusion was 5 minutes after infusion.[30] The primary target of SnET2 phototoxicity may be the endothelial cell.[31] It induces cell membrane damage and inhibits membrane transport by lipid peroxidation with singlet oxygen.[27,32] This photodamage is associated with significant membrane depolarization and opening of ion channels, increasing ion transport and decreasing amino acid uptake into the cell. This leads to endothelial cell damage, the release of thromboxanes, and vascular stasis.[33]

Ocular toxicity was transient and appeared confined to the RPE and outer photoreceptors. In a rabbit model,[29] histological studies performed after infusion of SnET2 at a dose of 0.5 mg/kg with light activation at a range of fluences from 5 J/cm² to 20 J/cm² yielded several findings. Retinal discoloration and neurosensory detachment were seen with the severity being dose-dependent. Subretinal fluid was present, especially in the areas of high irradiation. The RPE cells were disrupted and the photoreceptors were detached with cellular vacuolization. Retinal vessels remained uninjured. All these injuries resolved completely by day 28.[29]

SnET2 has been associated with cutaneous toxicity. In a murine model,[34] doses greater than 2.0 mg/kg resulted in significant skin damage in all test subjects. This was presumed to be due to the lingering presence of the photosensitizer in the plasma and skin. In phase I and II studies for the treatment of cutaneous cancers using 0.1 to 1.6 mg/kg doses of SnET2, 10% of patients experienced a mild transient sun sensitivity that lasted up to 1 month.[35] Aside from this transient sun sensitivity, SnET2 was well tolerated.

The results of a Phase III clinical trial investigating the usefulness of SnET2 for the treatment of classic choroidal neovascularization were pending at the time of this book's publication.

LUTETIUM TEXAPHYRIN

Lutetium texaphyrin is a pure, chemically stable, water-soluble photosensitizer with a bimodal absorption peak centered at 474 and 732 nm.[8,20,36-38] The 732-nm wavelength is preferable for use in PDT as the longer wavelength provides deeper penetration into the retina. Significant properties include increased solubility, deeper tissue penetration of the activating light, and minimal toxicity.[5,37,39,40] Most importantly, lutetium texaphyrin forms long-lived triplet states with efficient production of singlet oxygen.[39,40]

Lutetium texaphyrin is dissolved in 5% mannitol and administered intravenously.[5,8,38,41] Plasma concentrations are directly related to the dose administered. Systemic plasma concentrations peak between 5 to 30 minutes after intravenous injections of up to 10 μmol/kg.[8] The photosensitizer is rapidly cleared from the plasma with no detectable levels at 24 hours.[5,38] There is substantial accumulation of the drug in the liver and kidney, with lower levels in the skin and muscle. Levels remain present in the renal and hepatic system 24 hours after photosensitizer injection despite complete plasma clearance.[13]

Peak plasma concentrations may also be extrapolated from studies using Lu-Tex (Alcon, Fort Worth, Tex) as a fluorescent agent during angiography. After intravenous injection of 2 to 3 mg/kg of Lu-Tex over 30 seconds, maximal fluorescence in the normal retinal vessels of a CNV model occurred at 30 to 90 seconds, faded rapidly, and was absent after 18 minutes. Fluorescent properties of the choroid and CNV mirrored one another with maximal fluorescence occurring at 1 minute, followed by a plateau from 10 to 45 minutes. The CNV displayed fluorescence up to 5 hours after injection.[36]

Preclinical studies investigating the effectiveness of lutetium texaphyrin as a photosensitizing agent for treatment of CNV were performed in a monkey model with experimentally induced CNV. Lutetium texaphyrin was injected intravenously at a dose of 1 to 2 mg/kg.

Irradiation of the CNV occurred with a fluence of 50 and 100 J/cm[2]. Neovascular endothelial damage and choriocapillaris occlusion occurred from 5 to 48 minutes after injection with the neurosensory retina sustaining only minimal damage. Injury to the normal retinal vasculature occurred only at the 2 mg/kg dose with a fluence of 100 J/cm[2].[42]

In a phase I clinical trial using lutetium texaphyrin as treatment for metastatic cancers to the skin, intravenous doses of 0.6 to 7.2 mg/kg were well tolerated. Toxicity at the 7.2 mg/kg dose included dysesthesia in light-exposed skin and pain in the treatment field. Sensitivity to light occurred in roughly 5% of the patients.[43] Nonhuman trials using similar intravenous doses of lutetium texaphyrin failed to elucidate any systemic toxicity. At a dose of 40 mg/kg, transient acceleration in heart rate, tachypnea, and tremors have been observed. The LD[90] has been reported at 100 mg/kg.[5] In phase II trials for the treatment of CNV, the photosensitizer was well tolerated at a dose of 2.0 mg/kg and fluences of 50, 60, and 95 J/cm[2]. Side effects included transient parasthesias of the fingertips and eye discomfort. There were no reported cases of skin toxicity (personal communication, Jim Weiss, Pharmacyclics, Inc, Sunnyvale, Calif).

An advantage of lutetium texaphyrin is its bimodal absorption bands with an emission spectrum centered at 750 nm. This enables lutetium texaphyrin to be used as both an angiographic imaging tool and photosensitizer.[8,36,43,44] Since the 732-nm wavelength is used for PDT, this is the preferred wavelength for angiography. Sodium fluorescein, lutetium texaphyrin, and indocyanine green were compared in experimentally induced retinal and choroidal lesions. Lutetium texaphyrin was found to have properties somewhere between fluorescein and indocyanine green, with a molecular weight and plasma protein binding properties more similar to indocyanine green.[8,44] Histological analysis of retina demonstrated no associated retinal toxicity when lutetium texaphyrin was used as an angiographic agent in the presence of the photography flash.[8,44]

ATX-S10(Na)

ATX-S10(Na) is a water-soluble, synthetic, chlorine-derived photosensitizing agent with an absorption peak at 670 nm.[18,19,45,46] It is administered as an intravenous bolus. In a rat model with a dose of 16 mg/kg, ATX-S10(Na) reached a maximum plasma concentration immediately following administration. It is rapidly excreted with a half-life of 45 minutes.[47] ATX-S10(Na) is highly conjugated with HDL and albumin in plasma with less than 3% existing in an unbound form.[48]

While the systemic biodistribution of ATX-S10(Na) has not been elucidated, the cellular uptake of ATX-S10(Na) appears to involve endocytosis with preferential accumulation in lysosomes.[18] After a dose of 16 mg/kg in Long-Evans rats,[46] peak concentration of the drug in the choroid, retinal vasculature, retina outer segment, and RPE was present from 5 to 30 minutes, with significantly diminished levels by 2 hours. However, the arterial wall of the choroid retained the photosensitizing dye for up to 6 hours after injection. In CNV, peak concentrations occurred between 30 minutes to 2 hours after administration. Levels of ATX-S10(Na) in the CNV were undetectable by 24 hours. The sclera retained high concentrations for up to 6 hours post-injection.

Selective CNV occlusion in rats was obtained after treatment with a dose of 16 mg/kg of ATX-S10(Na). The ability to induce closure of the CNV persisted for up to 4 hours after injection.[46] Damage to the choriocapillaris and endothelium with increased platelet adhesion to the choroidal vessel endothelium was noted. In rats using a dose of 8 mg/kg of ATX-S10(Na) and fluences of 7.4 and 19.6 J/cm[2], successful CNV closure for a period of 28 days was obtained. Histological damage to the choriocapillaris, RPE cells, and photoreceptors was observed.[31] In monkey eyes, selective CNV closure for up to 28 days occurred after an 8 mg/kg dose of ATX-S10(Na).[18] Histological examination of the treated eyes demonstrated damage to the choriocapillaris, RPE, and outer photoreceptor segments. Recovery of the choriocapillaris occurred within 1 week, while the RPE and photoreceptor damage persisted.

CHLOROALUMINUM SULFONATED PHTHALOCYANINE (CASPC)

Chloroaluminum sulfonated phthalocyanine (CASPc) is a water-soluble, synthetic porphyrin sensitizer in the phthalocyanine (PC) group. A hydrophilic compound with an average of three sulfonic acid groups per molecule,[11,13,15] CASPc has a strong absorption peak at 675 nm.[11] The addition of the dimagnetic metal aluminum to the PC sensitizer extends the lifetime of its triplet state and reduces its tendency to aggregate in water, enhancing phototoxicity.[11,12,14]

In animal studies, CASPc reached peak serum levels immediately following injection.[11,49] Levels in serum and urine dramatically decrease after 2 days, though low levels can be detected in the serum for 8 days.[49,50] The water solubility of CASPc facilitates rapid excretion,[15] which occurs primarily by the renal system with some delayed excretion in feces.[51] There is no significant metabolism of the photosensitizing agent prior to excretion.

Systemic toxicity appears to be negligible as there have been no reported side effects in mice, guinea pigs, rabbits, cats, and dogs in doses as high as 100 mg/kg.[49-53] Skin toxicity with CASPc was found to be low in mice and highly dose-dependent.[11,54,55] In guinea pigs, it produced only minor skin sensitivity.[56]

Studies by Puliafito and associates in 1989 using CASPc to treat experimental CNV in monkeys validated the concept of photodynamic therapy for CNV.

The mechanism for localization of PC photosensitizers in neovascular tissue is poorly defined.[10,16] One method may occur by simple extravasation of the drug through leaky vasculature. Utilization of the lipoprotein pathway is another proposed mechanism, where proliferating endothelial cells demonstrate increased LDL receptors with receptor-mediated endocytosis.[56] Regardless of the mechanism, studies with experimental CNV in cynomolgus monkeys[17] demonstrated that CASPc localized in experimentally induced CNV for a period of 24 hours after a bolus infusion of 3 mg/kg. Treatment initiated 5 to 30 minutes after a 3 mg/kg intravenous dose of CASPc with 5 mW for 2 minutes produced closure of the CNV. Transient serous retinal detachments were noted clinically. Histological studies revealed vacuolization of the outer retina with minimal photoreceptor damage.[17]

MONO-L-ASPARTYL CHLORIN E6 (NPE6)

Mono-L-Aspartyl Chlorin e6 (NPe6) is a potent, hydrophilic, second-generation photosensitizer with an absorption peak at 664 nm.[53] Due to its hydrophilic nature, NPe6 is available in an aqueous preparation suitable for rapid infusion.[57] In mouse studies,[58] NPe6 reached peak serum concentration from 2 to 60 minutes after bolus infusion. Twenty-four hours after administration, highest tissue concentrations of NPe6 were identified in the liver, kidney, and spleen with trace concentrations present in skin, brain, and muscle. In vitro studies suggest that cellular uptake occurs through endocytosis.[59] NPe6 undergoes minimal metabolic transformation and is excreted primarily via the hepatic system.[58]

Histological analyses of monkey eyes suggest that PDT with NPe6 induces minimal local toxicity.[57] NPe6 phototoxicity occurs via destruction of the lysosome[59] and induced collateral damage primarily to the endothelial cells of the choriocapillaris and RPE cells at a dose of 10 mg/kg. Some larger choroidal vessels were occluded in addition to the choriocapillaris. There were few alterations in the inner retina aside from shortening of some outer segments with retinal vessels remaining unchanged.

CONCLUSION

Research continues to develop new photosensitizing agents that more closely match the profile of an ideal photosensitizer. The newer agents are highly photosensitive with long absorption wavelengths. Benzoporphyrin derivative has been proven effective relative to placebo in a large, randomized, multicenter clinical trial.[6] Tin etiopurpurin dichloride is currently undergoing similar scrutiny in clinical trials. A more recent photosensitizer, lutetium texaphyrin, may offer the benefit of a combination PDT/angiographic agent. Lutetium texaphyrin, NPe6, and the newer photosensitizer ATX-S10(Na) are hydrophilic compounds exhibiting rapid delivery to target tissue, high tissue concentrations, and prompt elimination. Side effect profiles appear very favorable with these newer compounds.

Considerations for future photosensitizing agents should incorporate the benefits of the current agents while optimizing selective accumulation in neovascular tissue and minimizing local and systemic toxicity. Another important issue involves the need for frequent retreatment due to reopening or recurrence of the choroidal neovascular complex. Future PDT agents will hopefully offer more permanent closure of CNV with a diminished need for retreatment. In the meantime, current photosensitizers permit an exciting new treatment alternative with advantages over conventional therapies such as laser photocoagulation.

REFERENCES

1. Freund KB, Yanuzzi LA, Sorenson JA. Age-related macular degeneration and choroidal neovascularization. *Am J Ophthalmol.* 1993;115:786-791.

2. Macular Photocoagulation Study Group. Argon laser photocoagulation for neovascular maculopathy: five-year results from randomized clinical trials. *Arch Ophthalmol.* 1991;109:1109-1114.

3. Macular Photocoagulation Study Group. Laser photocoagulation of subfoveal neovascular lesions in age-related macular degeneration: results of a randomized clinical trial. *Arch Ophthalmol.* 1991;109:1220-1231.

4. Dougherty TJ, Marcus SL. Photodynamic therapy. *Eur J Cancer.* 1992;28A:1734-1742.

5. Hammer-Wilson MJ, Ghahramanlou M, Berns MW. Photodynamic activity of lutetium-texaphyrin in a mouse tumor system. *Lasers Surg Med.* 1999;24:276-284.

6. Treatment of Age-Related Macular Degeneration with Photodynamic Therapy (TAP) Study Group. Photodynamic therapy of subfoveal choroidal neovascularization in age-related macular degeneration with verteporfin: one-year results of 2 randomized clinical trials—TAP report 1. *Arch Ophthalmol.* 1999;117:1329-1345.

7. Roberts WG, Hasan T. Role of neovasculature permeability on the tumor retention of photodynamic agents. *Cancer Res.* 1992;52:924-930.

8. Blumenkrantz MS, Woodburn KW, Qing F, et al. Lutetium texaphyrin (Lu-Tex): a potential new agent for ocular fundus angiography and photodynamic therapy. *Am J Ophthalmol.* 2000;129:353-362.

9. Henderson BW, Donovan JM. Release of prostaglandin E2 from cells by photodynamic treatment in vitro. *Cancer Res.* 1989;49:6896-6900.

10. Rutledge J, Curry F, Blanche P, et al. Solvent drag of LDL across mammalian endothelial barriers with increased permeability. *Am J Physiol.* 1995;268:H1982-H1991.

11. Bown SG, Tralau PD, Smith D. Photodynamic therapy with porphyrin and phthalocyanines sensitization: quantitative studies in normal rat liver. *Br J Cancer.* 1986;54:43-52.

12. Rosenthal I, Ben Hur E. Phthalocyanines in photobiology. In: Lever APB, Leznoff CC, eds. *Phthalocyanines, Properties and Applications.* New York, NY: VCH Publishers;1989:395-425.

13. Tralau CJ, MacRobert AJ, Coleridge-Smith PD, et al. Photodynamic therapy with phthalocyanine sensitization: quantitative studies in transplantable rat fibrosarcoma. *Br J Cancer.* 1987;55:389-395.

14. Moan J, Peng Q, Evensen JF, et al. Photosensitizing efficiencies, tumor and cellular uptake of different photosensitizing drugs relevant for photodynamic therapy of cancer. *Photochem Photobiol.* 1987;46:713-721.

15. Rosenthal I. Phalocyanines as photosensitizers. *Photochem Photobiol.* 1991;53:859-870.

16. Henderson BW, Dougherty TJ. How does photodynamic therapy work? *Photochem Photobiol.* 1992;55:145-157.

17. Kliman GH, Puliafito CA, Stern D, et al. Phthalocyanine photodynamic therapy: new strategy for closure of choroidal neovascularization. *Lasers Surg Med.* 1994;15:2-10.

18. Obana A, Gohto Y, Kanai M, et al. Selective photodynamic effects of the new photosensitizer ATX-S10(Na) on choroidal neovascularization in monkeys. *Arch Ophthalmol.* 2000;118:650-658.

19. Roberts WG, Smith M, McCullough JL, Berns MW. Skin photosensitivity and photodestruction of several potential photodynamic sensitizers. *Photochem Photobiol.* 1989;49:431-438.

20. Rivellese MJ, Baumal CR. Photodynamic therapy of eye diseases. *Ophth Surg Lasers.* 1999;30:653-661.

21. Allison BA, Pritchard PH, Richter AM, et al. The plasma distribution of benzoporphyrin derivative and the effects of plasma lipoproteins on its biodistribution. *Photochem Photobiol.* 1990;52:501-507.

22. Allison BA, Waterfield E, Richter AM, et al. The effects of plasma lipoproteins on in vitro tumor cell killing and in vivo tumor photosensitization with benzoporphyrin derivative. *Photochem Photobiol.* 1991;54:709-715.

23. Harriman A, Maiya BG, Hemmi T, et al. Met alotexaphyrins: a new family of photosensitizers for efficient generation of singlet oxygen. *J Chem Soc Chem Commun.* 1989;5:314-316.

24. Husain D, Miller JW, Michaud N, et al. Intravenous infusion of liposomal benzoporphyrin derivative for photodynamic therapy of experimental choroidal neovascularization. *Arch Ophthalmol.* 1996;114:978-985.

25. Ricchelli F, Barbato P, Milani M, et al. Photophysical properties of porphyrin plana aggregates in liposomes. *Eur J Biochem.* 1998;253:760-765.

26. Husain D, Kramer M, Kenny AG, et al. Effects of photodynamic therapy using verteporfin on experimental choroidal neovascularization and normal retina and choroids up to 7 weeks after treatment. *Invest Ophthalmol Vis Sci.* 1999;40:2322-2331.

27. Kessel D. Determinants of photosensitization by purpins. *Photochem Photobiol.* 1989;50:169-174.

28. Garbo GM. Purpurins and benzochlorins as sensitizers for photodynamic therapy. *J Photochem Photobio.* 1996;34:109-116.

29. Peyman G, Moshfeghi DM, Moshfeghi A, et al. Photodynamic therapy for choriocapillaris using tin ethyl etiopurpin (SnET2). *Ophthalmic Surg Lasers.* 1997;28:409-417.

30. Moshfeghi DM, Peyman GA, Moshfeghi A, et al. Ocular vascular thrombosis following tin ethyl etiopurpurin (SnET2) photodynamic therapy: time dependencies. *Ophthalmic Surg Lasers.* 1998;29:663-668.

31. Kessel D, Morgan A, Garbo GM. Sites and efficacy of photodamage by tin etiopurpurin in vitro using different delivery systems. *Photochem Photobiol.* 1991;54:193-196.

32. Morgan A, Cheng LD, Skalkos D, et al. Tin etiopurpurin dichloride-sensitized lipid photooxidation of erythrocyte membranes. *Photochem Photobiol.* 1990;52:987-991.

33. He DP, Hampton JA, Keck R, et al. Photodynamic therapy: effect on the endothelial cell of the rat aorta. *Photochem Photobiol.* 1991;54:801-804.

34. Morgan AR, Garbo GM, Keck RW, et al. Metallopurpurins and light: effect on transplantable rat bladder tumors and murine skin. *Photochem Photobiol.* 1990;51:589-592.

35. Razum NJ, Snyder AB, Doiron DR. SnET2: clinical update. *SPIE Proceedings.* 1996;2675:43-46.

36. Graham KB, Arbour JD, Connolly EJ, et al. Digital angiography using lutetium texaphyrin in a monkey model of choroidal neovascularization. *Invest Ophthalmol Vis Sci.* 1999;40:S402.

37. Grossweiner LI, Bilgin MD, Berdusis P, et al. Singlet oxygen generation by met allotexaphyrins. *Photochem Photobiol.* 1999;70:138-145.

38. Woodburn KW, Fan Q, Miles DR, et al. Localization and efficacy analysis of the phototherapeutic lutetium texaphyrin (PCI-0123) in the murine EMT6 sarcoma model. *Photochem Photobiol.* 1997;65:410-415.

39. Harriman A, Maiya BG, Hemmi T, et al. Metalotexaphyrins: a new family of photosensitizers for efficient generation of singlet oxygen. *J Chem Soc Chem Commun.* 1989;5:314-316.

40. Hill RA, Garrett J, Reddi S, et al. Photodynamic therapy (PDT) of the ciliary body with silicon naphthalcyanine (SINc) in rabbits. *Lasers Surg Med.* 1996;18:86-91.

41. Woodburn K, Fan Q, Kessel D, et al. Photodynamic therapy of B16F10 murine melanoma with lutetium texaphyrin. *J Invest Dermatol.* 1998;110:746-751.

42. Arbour JD, Connolly EJ, Graham K, et al. Photodynamic therapy of experimental choroidal neovascularization in a monkey model using intravenous infusion of lutetium texaphyrin. *Invest Ophthalmol Vis Sci.* 1991;40:S401.

43. Renschler MF, Yuen A, Panella TJ, et al. Photodynamic therapy trials with lutetium texaphyrin PC-0123 (Lu-Tex). *Photochem Photobiol.* 1997;65:46S.

44. Blumenkrantz MS, Woodburn K, Verdooner S. Lutetium texaphyrin angiography: a new method for the evaluation and treatment of retinal and choroidal vascular disorders. *Invest Ophthalmol Vis Sci.* 1988;39:S468.

45. Kanai M, Obana A, Gohto Y, et al. Long-term effectiveness of photodynamic therapy by using a hydrophilic photosensitizer ATX-S10(Na) against experimental choroidal neovascularization in rats. *Lasers Surg Med.* 2000;26:48-57.

46. Obana O, Gohto Y, Kaneda K, et al. Selective occlusion of choroidal neovascularization of photodynamic therapy with a water-soluble photosensitizer, ATX-S10. *Lasers Surg Med.* 1999;24:209-222.

47. Gohto Y, Obana A, Miki T. Photodynamic effect of a new photosensitizer ATX-S10 on corneal neovascularization. *Exp Eye Res.* 1988;67:313-322.

48. Mori M, Sakata A, Hirano T, et al. Photodynamic therapy for experimental tumors using ATX-S10(Na), a hydrophilic chlorin photosensitizer, and diode laser. *Jpn J Cancer Res.* 2000;91:753-759.

49. Tsilimbaris MK, Pallikaris I, Vlahonikolis IG, et al. Phthalocyanine mediated photodynamic thrombosis of experimental corneal neovascularization: effect of phthalocyanine dose and irradiation onset time on vascular occlusion rate. *Lasers Surg Med.* 1994;15:19-31.

50. Chan W, Marshall JF, Lam GYF, et al. Tissue uptake, distribution, and potency of the photoactivatable dye chloroaluminum sulfonated phthalocyanine in mice bearing transplantable tumors. *Cancer Research.* 1988;48:3040-3044.

51. Weintraub H, Abramovici A, Altman A, et al. Toxicity, tissue distribution and excretion studies of aluminum phthalocyanine tetrasulfate in normal mice. *Lasers Life Sci.* 1988;2:185-196.

52. Kliman GH, Puliafito CA, Grossman GA, et al. Retinal and choroidal vessel closure using phthalocyanine photodynamic therapy. *Lasers Surg Med.* 1994;15:11-18.

53. Roberts WG, Liaw LHL, Berns MW. In vitro photosensitization II. An electron microscopy study of cellular destruction with mono-l-aspartyl chlorin e6 and photofrin II. *Lasers Surg Med.* 1989;9:102-110.

54. Milanesi C, Biolo R, Reddi E, et al. Ultrastructural studies on the mechanism of the photodynamic therapy of tumors. *Photochem Photobiol.* 1987;46:675-681.

55. Tralau C, Young AR, Walker NPJ, et al. Mouse skin photosensitivity with dihaematoporphyrin ether (DHE) and aluminum sulfonated phthalocyanine (ALSPc): a comparative study. *Photochem Photobiol.* 1989;49:305-312.

56. Schmidt-Erfurth U, Hasan T, Gragoudas E, et al. Vascular targeting in photodynamic occlusion of subretinal vessels. *Ophthalmology.* 1994;106:1608-1614.

57. Mori K, Yonega S, Masataka O, et al. Angiographic and histological effects of fundus photodynamic therapy with a hydrophilic sensitizer (mono-l-aspartyl chlorin e6). *Ophthalmology.* 1999;106:1384-1391.

58. Gomer C, Ferrario A. Tissue distribution and photosensitizing properties of mono-l-aspartyl chlorin e6 in a mouse tumor model. *Cancer Res.* 1990;50:3985-3990.

59. Roberts WG, Berns MW. In vitro photosensitization I. Cellular uptake and subcellular localization of mono-l-aspartyl chlorin e6, chloro-aluminum sulfonated phthalocyanine, and photofrin II. *Lasers Surg Med.* 1989;9:90-101.

CHAPTER SIX

CLINICAL TRIALS FOR PHOTODYNAMIC THERAPY OF SUBFOVEAL CHOROIDAL NEOVASCULARIZATION

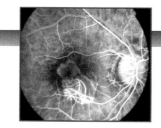 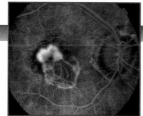 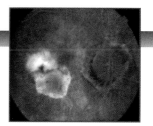

CHAPTER SECTIONS

INTRODUCTION

Subfoveal choroidal neovascularization (CNV) in patients with age-related macular degeneration (AMD) and pathologic myopia has been associated with poor visual outcomes. Prior to photodynamic therapy (PDT) with verteporfin, the only proven treatment modality for subfoveal CNV was laser photocoagulation. The Macular Photocoagulation Study[1-4] (MPS) examined the relative value of conventional laser ablation over observation for subfoveal CNV secondary to AMD. While some statistically significant visual benefits were reported, they were modest and not realized until 2 years after treatment. In addition, since subfoveal ablation causes acute visual loss relative to natural history in the short-term, many practitioners are hesitant to employ this treatment modality, reasoning that the modest long-term benefit may not justify the short-term irreversible visual loss. High recurrence rates after laser photocoagulation are also discouraging. Finally, the MPS results are not applicable to patients with poorly defined subfoveal CNV or CNV due to other causes such as pathologic myopia or ocular histoplasmosis syndrome (OHS). These limitations have prompted a search for improved therapeutic modalities for patients with subfoveal CNV. The Treatment of Age-Related Macular Degeneration with Photodynamic Therapy (TAP) Study Group[5,6] and the Verteporfin in Photodynamic Therapy (VIP) Study Group[7-9] conducted randomized, prospective, placebo-controlled trials evaluating PDT for the treatment of subfoveal CNV in patients with AMD and myopia. This chapter will briefly review the design, outcomes (Table 6-1), and limitations of these trials.

AGE-RELATED MACULAR DEGENERATION

Classic Choroidal Neovascularization: TAP Reports #1 & #2[5,6]

Design

The TAP Study enrolled 609 patients with subfoveal CNV secondary to AMD from multiple centers. Patients were assigned in a double-blind fashion to treatment with verteporfin (n = 402) or placebo (n = 207) (Figure 6-1). Eligible patients had a best-corrected ETDRS (Early Treatment Diabetic Retinopathy Study) visual acuity between 20/40 and 20/200 and subfoveal CNV due to AMD. The subfoveal CNV had to have a classic component (Figure 6-2). The size of the entire neovascular complex was limited to 5400 microns in the greatest linear dimension (9 MPS disc areas). The main outcome measured by the study was moderate visual loss defined as 3 ETDRS visual acuity lines. This represented a loss of 15 letters or a halving of the visual angle (eg, 20/80 to 20/160). At 24 months follow-up, outcomes were reported on 351 (87%) patients in the verteporfin group and 178 (86%) in the placebo group.

Outcomes

The primary outcome parameter was moderate visual loss. At 24 months, a statistically significant visual benefit was identified for a subgroup of patients with predominantly classic CNV (n = 159), defined as a lesion with a classic component occupying greater than or equal to 50% of the entire CNV complex (Figure 6-3). The remaining area of the lesion could consist of pigment epithelial detachment/occult CNV or blocked fluorescence from hemorrhage or other cause. At 2 years, moderate visual loss occurred in 41% of patients with predominantly classic membranes (n = 159) treated with verteporfin compared to 69%

TABLE 6-1						
TAP AND VIP STUDY OUTCOMES[5-8]						
Clinical Trial	**Study Parameters**	**<3 lines or 15 letters lost (%)**	**Initial VA (mean)**	**Final VA (mean)**	**VA <20/200 (%)**	**>6 lines or 30 letters lost (%)**
TAP	1 Year					
	Placebo	46	20/100	20/200	48	24
	Verteporfin	61	20/100	20/160	35	15
	2 Years					
	Placebo	38	20/100	20/200	55	30
	Verteporfin	53	20/100	20/160	41	18
VIP #1^	1 Year					
	Placebo	87	20/64	20/80**	26	8
	Verteporfin	67	20/64	20/64**	8	7
VIP #2*	1 Year					
	Placebo	54	20/50	20/126	32	33
	Verteporfin	49	20/50	20/100	20	22
	2 Years					
	Placebo	31	20/50	20/160	45	47
	Verteporfin	45	20/50	20/126	28	29

VA = visual acuity

^Primary outcome in VIP Report #1 was a 1.5-line visual loss or 8 letters

*Results from VIP Report #2 subgroup evaluating lesions with occult, but no classic

**VIP Report #1 reported median visual acuity

Note: >3-line loss is moderate visual loss, and >6-line loss is severe visual loss. The primary goal of the TAP and VIP trials was the prevention of moderate visual loss.

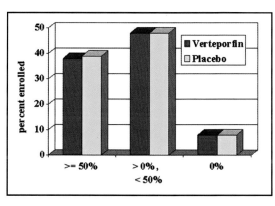

Figure 6-1. Initial enrollment in the TAP Study Group divided into subgroups based on the percentage of classic component of the CNV.[5,6]

Figure 6-2. Early (A) and late (B) fluorescein angiography of CNV with a classic and occult component.

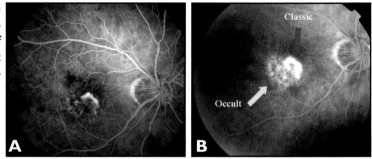

Figure 6-3. Percentage of eyes with moderate visual loss comparing verteporfin to placebo. Lesions containing 50% or more classic component benefited from treatment at the 1- and 2-year results. The number of patients without a classic component were not sufficient to provide a statistically significant result.[5,6]

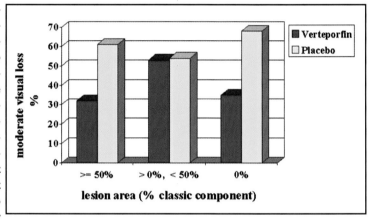

Figure 6-4. Graph demonstrating that predominantly classic lesions prevented moderate visual loss at both 12 and 24 months.[5,6]

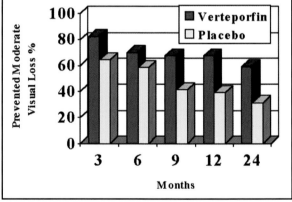

treated with placebo (n = 83) (Figure 6-4). Severe visual loss (loss of 6 or more lines) occurred in 15% of treated patients versus 36% of controls; legal blindness was present in 44% of treated patients versus 68% of controls (Figure 6-5). Both of these outcomes were statistically significant. Final visual acuity was not reported for this subgroup of patients with severe visual loss, though verteporfin-treated patients in general had a mean visual acuity of 20/160 compared to 20/200 in the control group at 2 years (Figures 6-6 and 6-7). Verteporfin-treated patients with predominantly classic CNV also demonstrated statistical-

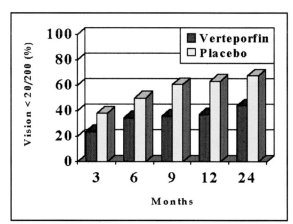

Figure 6-5. Percentage of eyes with visual acuity less than 20/200, comparing placebo with verteporfin-treated eyes.[5,6]

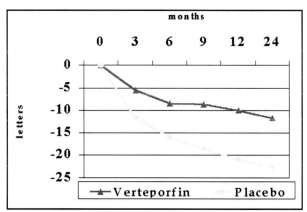

Figure 6-6. Two-year results of visual acuity comparing placebo with verteporfin.[5,6]

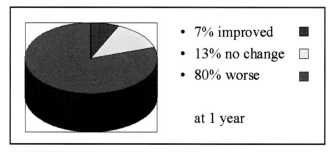

- 7% improved
- 13% no change
- 80% worse

at 1 year

Figure 6-7a. Comparison of visual acuity of eyes treated with placebo.[5,6]

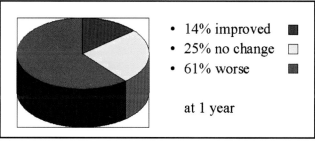

- 14% improved
- 25% no change
- 61% worse

at 1 year

Figure 6-7b. Comparison of visual acuity of eyes treated with verteporfin.[5,6]

Figure 6-8. Results of contrast sensitivity testing in eyes treated with verteporfin and with placebo.[5,6]

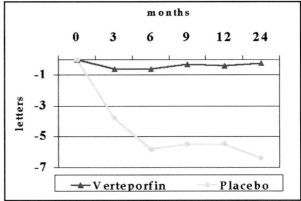

Figure 6-9. Graph demonstrating that verteporfin induces more complete and partial closure of CNV compared to placebo.[5,6]

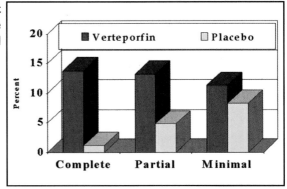

Figure 6-10. One year following treatment, verteporfin-treated lesions are considerably smaller than placebo-treated eyes.[5,6]

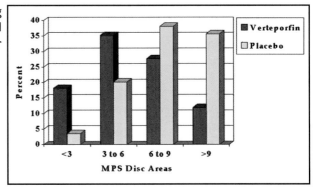

ly significant benefits in preserving contrast sensitivity and fluorescein angiographic outcomes, including limiting progression to classic CNV, absence of leakage, and decreased final lesion size (Figures 6-8 through 6-10).

Retreatment was documented for both study groups. In the first year, there was an average of 3.4 treatments in the verteporfin group compared to 3.7 treatments in the placebo group. This decreased to 2.1 for the second year in the verteporfin group. Thus, the verteporfin-treated group averaged 5.5 treatments over 2 years. It is important to understand that subgroup analysis for retreatment of predominantly classic lesions was not performed.

Occult Choroidal Neovascularization: VIP Report #2[7]

Design

The second VIP Report focused primarily on patients with occult subfoveal CNV without any classic component. Two hundred-twenty-five eyes were in the treatment group and 114 were in the control group. Eligibility requirements included lesion size less than 5400 microns and visual acuity of at least 20/100. Occult lesions were required to have associated hemorrhage or deterioration within 3 months of enrollment. Deterioration was defined as loss of 1 ETDRS visual acuity line or an increase in the lesion's greatest linear dimension by 10%.

Outcomes

At 1 year, no statistically significant differences were found between the verteporfin-treated patients and controls with respect to reducing risk of moderate and severe visual loss. At 2 years, however, a statistically significant difference was found: 54% of verteporfin-treated eyes compared to 67% of controls experienced moderate visual loss. Mean final visual acuity was 20/126 in the verteporfin-treated eyes and 20/160 in the control eyes. Severe visual loss occurred in 30% of verteporfin-treated eyes compared to 46% of controls; in addition, 28% of verteporfin-treated eyes compared to 45% of controls were legally blind. Both of these outcomes were statistically significant.

Four percent of verteporfin-treated eyes experienced acute visual loss defined as at least 20 letters within 7 days of treatment. This phenomenon was not observed in controls. Etiologies included hemorrhagic pigment epithelial detachment, neurosensory detachment, and idiopathic visual loss.

Conclusions

The TAP Study demonstrated that verteporfin is effective in reducing moderate visual loss for predominantly classic subfoveal CNV secondary to AMD. However, these results must be evaluated in light of several possible shortcomings in study design. Patients with subfoveal CNV in the placebo group were observed instead of being treated per MPS guidelines. Other studies, such as the Submacular Surgery Trial[10] (SST), have used foveal laser photocoagulation as a control. Double-blinding in the TAP Study, however, would not have been possible if the control group had received laser photocoagulation. In contrast, double-blinding in the SST was never an option due to the surgical intervention in the study group. Interpretation of results with PDT relative to placebo must take into account the possible benefit that conventional laser photocoagulation may have had in this study population. One may even question if a statistically significant benefit would have been achieved since both treatment modalities demonstrated a modest benefit over the natural history of untreated subfoveal CNV secondary to AMD.

The finding of efficacy only in the predominantly classic subgroup invites further criticism. The concept of subgroups was not introduced at study enrollment, at which time only the presence of a classic component was required. A pure prospective study tests a hypothesis on a predetermined study population and reports data on this population. To eliminate statistical confounding, subgroups should be specified prior to enrollment. The number of participants in each subgroup must also be determined in advance to enhance validity and help to achieve statistical significance for an effective intervention. One can argue that the TAP Study presented subgroup data that was retrospectively introduced into a prospective design. However, the study population was large enough to achieve statistical significance in the predominantly classic subgroup.

The TAP and VIP trials, like many studies on the treatment of CNV, documented visual and anatomic success. However, incremental improvements in acuity may have statistical but only limited clinical significance. The visual outcome from neovascular AMD tends to be disappointing regardless of intervention. This is reflected by the high rate of visual loss and legal blindness in both treatment and control groups. For example, the VIP Study Group recommended PDT for occult subfoveal CNV showing recent disease progression. However, no treatment benefit was realized at 1 year, and only a modest visual benefit was achieved after 2 years of follow-up. Incorporating functional data such as the National Eye Institute Visual Functioning Questionnaire (VFQ-25) may have further defined the actual clinical benefits of PDT for CNV.

Like the MPS, both trials are limited by patient eligibility requirements. For example, the TAP Study is more restrictive in terms of lesion components, while the MPS is more restrictive in terms of lesion size. A great majority of subfoveal neovascular lesions will fail to qualify for either treatment modality. Similarly, many occult lesions do not harbor a hemorrhagic component, nor do they progress over 3 months; these lesions fail to qualify under VIP #2 guidelines.

SUBFOVEAL CHOROIDAL NEOVASCULARIZATION FROM PATHOLOGIC MYOPIA

VIP Report #1

Design

The VIP Study on pathologic myopia enrolled 120 patients with subfoveal CNV, 81 in the treatment group and 39 in the control group. Eligibility requirements included 6.0 or more diopters of myopia or evidence of pathologic myopia with axial length of 26.5 mm or greater, a lesion size with a greatest linear dimension of 5400 microns, and a best-corrected visual acuity of 20/100 or better. On fluorescein angiography, the CNV could be classic or occult, and it had to be identifiable in at least 50% of the lesion's total area. Similar to the TAP Study, patients were eligible for retreatment at 3 months. The primary outcome measure was 8 letters or approximately 1.5 lines of visual acuity loss.

Outcomes

The verteporfin-treated patients had statistically significant reduction in visual loss compared to the placebo group at 12 months. Seventy-two percent of patients treated with verteporfin lost fewer than 8 letters of visual acuity compared to 44% of patients in the control group. The median visual acuity was 20/64+2 in the treatment group and 20/80-2 in the control group. The treatment group also had statistically significant improvements in contrast sensitivity relative to the controls. Patients received an average of 3.4 treatments during the year.

Conclusions

The VIP trial demonstrated that pathologic myopes with CNV had a statistically significant reduction in visual loss compared to the placebo group when treated with PDT using verteporfin. These results must be balanced against two limitations. First, the visual acuity eligibility requirements of 20/100 or better would exclude a large number of patients. Second, while a difference of 8 letters of visual loss between the treatment and control groups was statistically significant, it is debatable whether this difference is clinically significant. These results would have much more value if a practical measure (eg, reading speed) was used to place them in a clinical context.

REFERENCES

1. Macular Photocoagulation Study Group. Laser photocoagulation of subfoveal neovascular lesions in age-related macular degeneration: results of a randomized clinical trial. *Arch Ophthalmol*. 1991;109:1220-1231.

2. Macular Photocoagulation Study Group. Laser photocoagulation of subfoveal recurrent neovascular lesions in age-related macular degeneration: results of a randomized clinical trial. *Arch Ophthalmol*. 1991;109:1232-1241.

3. Macular Photocoagulation Study Group. Recurrent choroidal neovascularization after argon laser photocoagulation for neovascular maculopathy. *Arch Ophthalmol*. 1986;104:503-512.

4. Macular Photocoagulation Study Group. Subfoveal neovascular lesions in age-related macular degeneration: guidelines for evaluation and treatment in the macular photocoagulation study. *Arch Ophthalmol*. 1991;109:1242-1257.

5. Treatment of Age-Related Macular Degeneration with Photodynamic Therapy (TAP) Study Group. Photodynamic therapy of subfoveal choroidal neovascularization in age-related macular degeneration with verteporfin. *Arch Ophthalmol*. 1999;117:1329-1345.

6. Treatment of Age-Related Macular Degeneration with Photodynamic Therapy (TAP) Study Group. Photodynamic therapy of subfoveal choroidal neovascularization in age-related macular degeneration with verteporfin: two-year results of 2 randomized clinical trials—TAP Report #2. *Arch Ophthalmol*. 2001;119:198-207.

7. Verteporfin in Photodynamic Therapy (VIP) Study Group. Verteporfin therapy of subfoveal choroidal neovascularization in age-related macular degeneration: two-year results of a randomized clinical trial including lesions with occult with no classic choroidal neovascularization—VIP Report #2. *Am J Ophthalmol*. 2001;131:541-560.

8. Verteporfin in Photodynamic Therapy (VIP) Study Group. Photodynamic therapy of subfoveal choroidal neovascularization in pathologic myopia with verteporfin: one-year results of a randomized clinical trial—VIP Report #1. *Ophthalmology*. 2001;108:841-852.

9. Submacular Surgery Trials Pilot Study Investigators. Submacular surgery trials randomized pilot trial of laser photocoagulation versus surgery for recurrent choroidal neovascularization secondary to age-related macular degeneration: I. Ophthalmic outcomes—Submacular Surgery Trials Pilot Study Report #1. *Am J Ophthalmol*. 2000;130:387-407.

CHAPTER SEVEN

TREATMENT PROTOCOL FOR PHOTODYNAMIC THERAPY OF CHOROIDAL NEOVASCULARIZATION WITH VERTEPORFIN

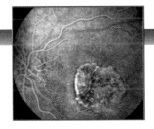 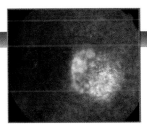 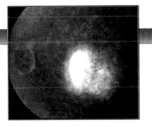

CHAPTER SECTIONS

Verteporfin is currently the only approved photosensitizer for the treatment of choroidal neovascularization (CNV) with photodynamic therapy (PDT). To utilize this treatment modality most safely and effectively, it is essential to understand the sequence of events in the treatment protocol. This chapter will review the case selection, treatment protocol, and postoperative care for PDT with verteporfin.

CASE SELECTION

Proper case selection for PDT with verteporfin involves a careful review of the indications and contraindications. Verteporfin is indicated for the treatment of predominantly classic subfoveal CNV due to age-related macular degeneration (AMD). This lesion type has shown a statistically significant benefit of treatment relative to placebo in a large, randomized, multicenter trial. Results of the Treatment of Age-Related Macular Degeneration with Photodynamic Therapy (TAP) Study[1,2] are reviewed in Chapter Six. Other etiologies of CNV are currently being studied in the Verteporfin in Photodynamic Therapy (VIP) Study,[3,4] and results are forthcoming.

Fluorescein angiography is required to document the choroidal neovascular complex with respect to lesion size, location, and components. The TAP Study restricted lesion size to 5400 microns (9 MPS disc areas) in the greatest linear dimension, although current PDT lasers are capable of producing larger spot sizes. The location of the lesion must involve the center of the foveal avascular zone. Finally, the lesion must contain a classic component that occupies at least 50% of the entire choroidal neovascular complex. Classic CNV was defined in the Macular Photocoagulation Study (MPS)[5] as a bright, uniform area of early hyperfluorescence that exhibits progressive leakage in the late phases (Figures 7-1 and 7-2). The remaining 50% of a qualifying PDT lesion may include pigment epithelial detachment (PED) and/or blocked fluorescence from hemorrhage or other cause. Prior laser photocoagulation scars are not included in the calculation, as they do not contribute to the active choroidal neovascular complex. Detailed angiographic interpretation is reviewed in Chapter Three.

Contraindications to PDT with verteporfin include pregnancy, liver disease, porphyria, or a known hypersensitivity to the photosensitizing agent (Table 7-1). The VIP Study Group reported that verteporfin was beneficial in the treatment of occult and myopic CNV.

INFORMED CONSENT

As with all interventional procedures, informed consent is required prior to PDT. The patient should understand the treatment procedure, the potential benefits of treatment, as well as possible adverse events. A sample procedure log (Figure 7-3) is shown that is currently being utilized at the New England Eye Center.

PREPARATION OF DRUG

PDT is a unique ophthalmic procedure in that it involves the intravenous administration of a photosensitizing agent. A skilled nurse is required to reduce the incidence of potentially devastating outcomes, such as improper dosage or extravasation.

Verteporfin is supplied as a lyophilized cake of 15 mg requiring reconstitution with 7 mL of sterile water (Figure 7-4). The resulting solution contains 15 mg in 7.5 mL or 2 mg/mL. After reconstitution, the drug should be protected from light and used within 4 hours.

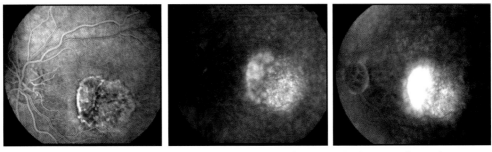

Figure 7-1. Fluorescein angiography demonstrating a lesion with classic and occult components; the occult component occupies greater than 50% of the entire lesion.

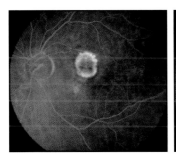
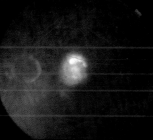

Figure 7-2. Fluorescein angiography demonstrating 100% classic CNV.

TABLE 7-1
CONTRAINDICATIONS TO PHOTODYNAMIC THERAPY

- Pregnancy
- Liver disease (a relative contraindication)
- Porphyria
- Known hypersensitivity to photosensitizing agent

The weight and height of the patient need to be measured. A nomogram is used to determine the body surface area (BSA). The BSA is required for proper dosage determination (Figure 7-5); a dosage of 6 mg/m^2 must be prepared. For example, a patient that has a BSA of 2 m^2 requires 12 mg of drug to be infused. Upon determining the milligram dosage, the volume of reconstituted verteporfin needs to be calculated. Since the solution contains 2 mg/mL, a simple conversion will yield the required value. In the example above, 12 mg of drug is contained in 6 mL of solution. The calculated drug volume is withdrawn into a separate syringe and diluted to a final volume of 30 mL using 5% dextrose. In the given example, 6 mL of solution would be diluted with 24 mL of 5% dextrose to yield a final volume of 30 mL. Proper dosing is essential since underdosage often results in inadequate treatment and overdosage can cause closure of larger retinal vessels with permanent visual loss.

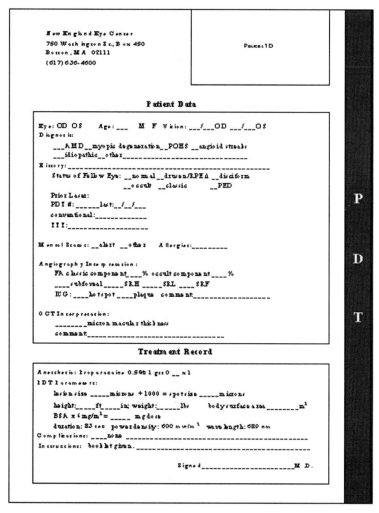

Figure 7-3. Sample procedure log.

LASER SETTINGS

Two laser devices (Figures 7-6 and 7-7) are currently approved for use in PDT with verteporfin: the Coherent Opal Photoactivator (Coherent, Santa Clara, Calif) and Zeiss Visulas 690s laser (Zeiss Humphrey Systems, Dublin, Calif). Both deliver stable power output at a wavelength of 689 nm. The light dose is 50 J/cm^2 or 600 mW/cm^2, which is automatically set by the photoactivator. Light energy is delivered over 83 seconds.

The laser devices require entry of a spot size to determine power density, as well as the magnification of the treatment lens. The Coherent Photoactivator stores magnifications of most commonly used lenses, which are summarized in Table 7-2.

The spot size is determined by evaluation of fluorescein angiography using a film-based or digital system. If a film-based system is used, spot size determination is performed by plac-

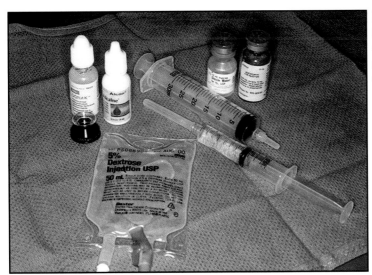

Figure 7-4. Basic set-up for preparation of verteporfin for infusion and treatment with PDT.

Step 1:	Determine body surface area (BSA) using nomogram
	(BSA = 2.0 m²)
Step 2:	Determine dosage in mg; required dosage is 6 mg/m²
	Dosage (mg) = 6 mg/m² x BSA (m²)
	(6 mg/m² x 2.0 m² = 12 mg)
Step 3:	Determine dosage of reconstituted verteporfin in mL; reconstituted to 2 mg/mL
	Dosage (mL) = Dosage (mg) ÷ 2 mg/mL
	(12 mg ÷ 2 mg/mL = 6 mL)
Step 4:	Dilute reconstituted dosage in mL to final volume of 30 mL
	30 mL − reconstituted dosage (mL) = dilution with 5% dextrose (mL)
	(30 mL − 6 mL = 24 mL)
	Dilute 6 mL reconstituted verteporfin with 24 mL 5% dextrose
Step 5:	Infuse diluted verteporfin over 10 minutes (3 mL/min)

Figure 7-5. Sample dosage calculation for PDT with verteporfin.

ing a supplied reticle over the choroidal neovascular complex that encompasses the greatest linear dimension (Figure 7-8). The magnification of the camera system must be known to determine the actual lesion size. For example, a lesion encompassed by a 5-mm reticle with a camera magnification of 2.5 has an actual dimension of 2 mm. If a digital system is utilized (Figure 7-9), most software programs offer a measuring function that can be used to determine lesion size. The cursor is dragged along the greatest linear dimension and the output is read from the screen. With either technique, care must be taken to include the greatest linear dimension of the entire neovascular complex. This includes all classic CNV, PED, and blocked fluorescence. Prior laser photocoagulation is not included in this measurement.

Figure 7-6. Coherent Opal Photoactivator (photo used with permission of Coherent, Inc, Santa Clara, Calif).

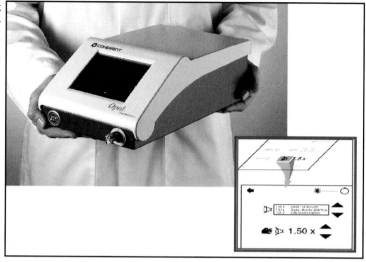

Figure 7-7. Zeiss Visulas 690s (photo used with permission of Zeiss Humphrey Systems, Dublin, Calif).

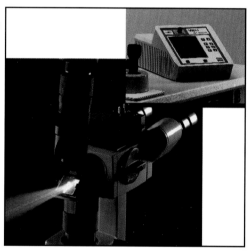

TABLE 7-2		

FUNDUS LENS MAGNIFICATIONS

Make	Model	Magnification
Volk	Area Centralis	1.04x
Ocular Instruments	Mainster Standard	1.05x
Ocular Instruments	3-Mirror Universal	1.08x
Volk	TransEquator	1.44x
Ocular Instruments	Mainster Widefield	1.50x
Volk	PDT	1.50x
Ocular Instruments	Mainster Ultrafield	1.90x
Volk	SupraQuad 160	1.92x
Volk	QuadraAspheric	2.01x

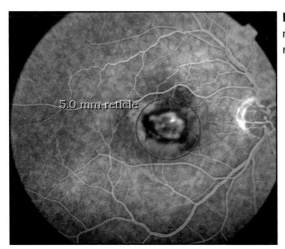

Figure 7-8. Sample spot size determination using film-based angiography and reticle.

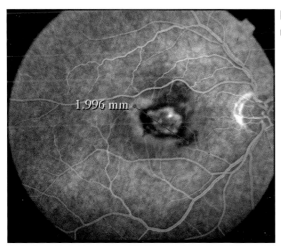

Figure 7-9. Sample spot size determination using digital angiography.

The final spot size is determined by adding 1000 microns to the greatest linear dimension (Figure 7-10). An untreated border of 200 microns is required temporal to the optic nerve head even if there is evidence of CNV in this location. Inadvertent treatment of the optic nerve head may result in optic neuropathy.

PHOTODYNAMIC THERAPY TREATMENT

PDT is a two-step procedure involving the intravenous administration of a photosensitizer followed by activation with a laser light source. Intravenous access is obtained by placing a 22-gauge catheter in an arm vein (Figure 7-11). The antecubital site is preferred to reduce the complication of extravasation from smaller, more fragile veins. An infusion pump is set to deliver 3 mL of solution per minute. The 30 mL is delivered over 10 minutes. The patient is monitored carefully during infusion. In the event of extravasation, the infusion should be stopped immediately. If less than half (15 mL) of the dose has been administered, better venous access should be obtained. The infusion should then be restarted and the

Figure 7-10. Sample final lesion size determination (greatest linear dimension + 1000 microns).

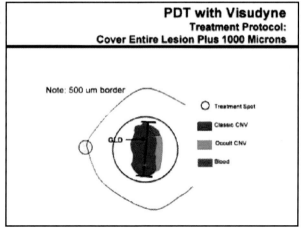

Figure 7-11. Infusion pump and insertion of catheter into antecubital site.

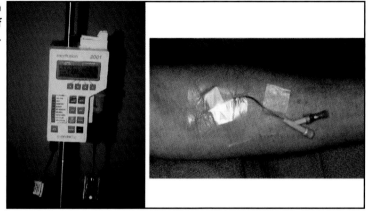

patient treated according to the protocol. If greater than half (15 mL) of the dose has been administered, treatment should proceed using the infused dose.

Laser treatment begins 15 minutes after the start of infusion (5 minutes after the completion of infusion). The spot size and treatment lens magnification should be entered into the photoactivator. The pupil should be widely dilated. Often, installation of additional dilating drops at the beginning of infusion will avoid the potential of pupillary constriction due to a lag between initial evaluation and treatment. Topical anesthetic drops are applied to the cornea, and the treatment lens is coupled to the cornea with methylcellulose gel. The patient is treated at the slit lamp for 83 seconds (Figure 7-12). It is helpful to have the angiogram available in the treatment room to view landmarks at the treatment borders and guide appropriate positioning of the spot. The patient is asked to look straight ahead and maintain fixation. Treatment may be suspended temporarily if there is excessive movement or refixation. Treatment proceeds until the 83-second interval expires.

PHOTOSENSITIVITY PRECAUTIONS

Special precautions are necessary after PDT with verteporfin and must be explained to each treated patient. Patients are advised to avoid direct sunlight for 5 days. All exposed

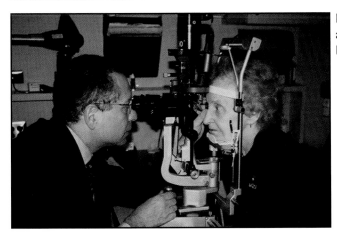

Figure 7-12. PDT performed at the slit lamp using a contact lens and topical anesthesia.

body surfaces should be protected in the event that it is necessary to go outdoors during daylight hours. Dark sunglasses, long sleeves, and a wide-brimmed hat are recommended. Additional light sources to avoid include tanning beds, bright halogen lights, and surgical or dental operative lights. It is important to understand that ultraviolet sunscreening products will not protect from photosensitivity since the drug is activated by light in the visible spectrum.

Follow-Up Care, Retreatment, and Bilateral Treatment

Patients should be warned of potential transient visual disturbance that often occurs shortly after treatment. This typically resolves within the first postoperative week. A small subset of patients (1% to 4%) will experience severe vision decrease defined as 4 or more lines within the first 7 days. Many of these patients experience partial recovery.

Patients should also be notified of the frequent need for retreatment. Follow-up is planned at 3-month intervals, at which time fluorescein angiography is repeated to evaluate response to treatment. The authors typically examine patients 1 month following treatment to evaluate their progress. If there is evidence of continued leakage from the neovascular complex, retreatment is planned according to the same protocol as initial treatment.

Bilateral treatment can be considered in patients with qualifying lesions in both eyes. It is recommended that the initial treatment be performed on one eye in case there is a significant negative outcome. After safely performing the procedure in one eye, the fellow eye can be treated 1 week later using the same protocol. On retreatment visits, bilateral treatment can be performed with a single infusion. The more aggressive lesion is treated first, 15 minutes after infusion. The laser parameters are reset for the second lesion and treatment can proceed no later than 20 minutes after infusion.

Adverse Events

Though PDT is generally a safe procedure, adverse effects have been observed (Table 7-3). The most serious adverse events are severe vision loss and extravasation of the photosensitizer.

In the event of severe vision loss (1% to 4% of patients), the patient is counseled and followed closely for recovery of lost vision. Retreatment is obviously not advisable. Partial

TABLE 7-3
ADVERSE EVENTS
• Visual disturbance (blurred vision, decreased acuity, visual field defect) • Injection site event (extravasation, rash) • Photosensitivity • Allergic reaction • Back pain • Headache

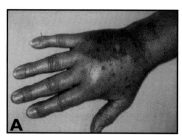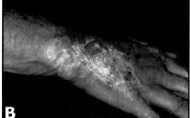

Figure 7-13. The verteporfin infusion site for this patient was at the wrist. There was no noticeable extravasation at the time of infusion. Within 24 hours, the hand and wrist were exposed to bright sunlight for several hours. The hand became swollen and painful. The patient was treated with cold compresses, analgesics, and a Medrol steroid dose pack. (A) Appearance of the hand 10 days after sun exposure with apparent swelling and discoloration of the skin. (B) Appearance of the hand 40 days after sun exposure with ulceration and necrosis consistent with a third-degree burn. The skin eventually healed after 90 days without the need for skin grafting. This is why all infusion sites must be protected from bright light exposure for at least 5 days (photos reprinted with permission from Philip Rosenfeld, MD and Novartis Ophthalmics, Bulach, Switzerland. © Novartis Ophthalmics).

recovery of vision is observed in many patients experiencing severe vision decrease, defined as 4 or more lines within 1 week of treatment.

In the event of extravasation, the affected area should be protected from light for a minimum of 2 days and as long as any discoloration of the skin is visible. A cold compress or ice should be applied immediately, and the arm elevated for 1 day. Pain medication should be prescribed as needed. Even if no extravasation occurs, the infusion site should be protected from light (Figure 7-13).

The most common adverse events in the TAP Study were visual disturbances and injection site events.[1] Headache was also a common complaint. Visual disturbance (including blurred vision, decreased visual acuity, and visual field defect) occurred in 17.7% of verteporfin-treated patients compared to 11.6% of placebo-treated patients. Injection site events (including extravasation and rash) occurred in 13.4% of verteporfin-treated patients

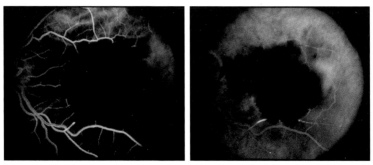

Figure 7-14. Fluorescein angiography 1 week following PDT with verteporfin. Treatment was performed using a light dose of 150 J/cm² applied 30 minutes after an infusion dose of 12 mg/m² during a phase I and II study. Macular infarction is present with nonperfusion of both the arterioles and venules. Standard PDT currently uses a light dose of 50 J/cm² with a verteporfin dose of 6 mg/m² (photos reprinted with permission from *Arch Ophthalmol.* 1999;117:1161-73. ©1999, American Medical Association).

compared to 3.4% of placebo-treated patients. Other adverse events included photosensitivity in 3% of patients, allergic reaction in 1.2% of patients, and back pain in 2.2% of patients.

Overdosage of the drug and/or light may cause nonperfusion of normal retinal vessels with subsequent severe visual loss from macular infarction (Figure 7-14).

REFERENCES

1. Treatment of Age-Related Macular Degeneration with Photodynamic Therapy (TAP) Study Group. Photodynamic therapy of subfoveal choroidal neovascularization in age-related macular degeneration with verteporfin. *Arch Ophthalmol.* 1999;117:1329-1345.

2. Treatment of Age-Related Macular Degeneration with Photodynamic Therapy (TAP) Study Group. Photodynamic therapy of subfoveal choroidal neovascularization in age-related macular degeneration with verteporfin: two-year results of 2 randomized clinical trials—TAP Report #2. In press.

3. Verteporfin in Photodynamic Therapy (VIP) Study Group. Photodynamic therapy of subfoveal choroidal neovascularization in pathologic myopia with verteporfin: one-year results of a randomized clinical trial—VIP Report #1. In press.

4. Verteporfin in Photodynamic Therapy (VIP) Study Group. Photodynamic therapy of subfoveal choroidal neovascularization in age-related macular degeneration with verteporfin: one-year results of a randomized clinical trial including lesions with occult but no classic neovascularization—VIP Report #2. In press.

5. Macular Photocoagulation Study Group. Subfoveal neovascular lesions in age-related macular degeneration: guidelines for evaluation and treatment in the macular photocoagulation study. *Arch Ophthalmol.* 1991;1242-1257.

CHAPTER EIGHT

PRACTICAL APPLICATIONS OF PHOTODYNAMIC THERAPY FOR CHOROIDAL NEOVASCULARIZATION

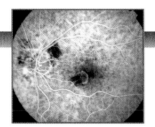 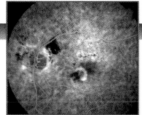 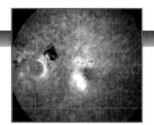

CHAPTER SECTIONS

❖ Photodynamic Therapy Classification System

❖ Applications of the Classification System

❖ Case Reports

❖ Summary

The Treatment of Age-Related Macular Degeneration with Photodynamic Therapy (TAP) Study Group confirmed photodynamic therapy (PDT) with verteporfin as a beneficial treatment option for predominantly classic, subfoveal choroidal neovascularization (CNV).[1] However, other factors appear to influence the efficacy of PDT in age-related macular degeneration (AMD). This chapter will review practical applications of this therapeutic modality in lesions that qualify for treatment by TAP Study criteria. Lesions will be further characterized to allow for selection of cases that will best respond to PDT in terms of both visual benefit and anatomic closure. In contrast, characteristics that impart a poorer prognosis will be discussed in defining the limitations of this new procedure. Through proper case selection, lesions may be treated in the safest and most efficacious manner. Patients can be better counseled regarding the expected outcome in their specific cases. The need for multiple retreatments, a common event in the TAP Study, may also be minimized.

PHOTODYNAMIC THERAPY CLASSIFICATION SYSTEM

To best understand the events that occur after PDT, a classification system was developed using clinical features and fluorescein angiography at specific time intervals after treatment. Optical coherence tomography (OCT) findings were incorporated since this technology provides anatomic cross-sectional data that accurately reflect the retinal status at specific post-treatment intervals. After analysis of numerous cases over the initial 3-month period and subsequent retreatment periods, consistent OCT patterns emerged. These patterns were studied, allowing for the formulation and validation of a useful five-stage classification system. The five stages in the classification system are as follows:
- Stage I: Acute inflammatory response
- Stage II: Resolution of subretinal fluid with choroidal hypoperfusion
- Stage III: Reaccumulation of subretinal fluid with choroidal reperfusion
- Stage IV: Subretinal fibrosis with persistent retinal fluid
- Stage V: Subretinal fibrosis with retinal atrophy

Each stage will be defined with respect to clinical, angiographic, and OCT features. The classification system will then be applied as a basis for making intelligent treatment decisions.

To initiate the photodynamic process, an intravenously injected photosensitizing agent accumulates in ocular neovascular tissue[2] and is activated by nonthermal, wavelength-specific light. The formation of singlet oxygen along with the production of hydroxyl radicals, peroxides, and superoxides are believed to play a primary role in PDT-mediated phototoxicity.[3-6] A local inflammatory response is incited,[7,8] and occlusion of the CNV occurs from damage to endothelial cells, platelet activation, and thrombus formation.[4]

Stage I: Acute Inflammatory Response

Immediately following PDT, both fluorescein angiography and OCT demonstrate an acute, local inflammatory response. This has been confirmed on OCT as early as 15 minutes following photoactivation. Within 1 hour post-treatment, fluorescein angiography shows relative hyperfluorescence of both the CNV and the treatment area. There is actually increased leakage of the CNV and surrounding treatment zone in the late frames. The OCT reveals increased accumulation of diffuse intraretinal fluid in the circular distribution of the treatment spot (Figure 8-1). This phenomenon may explain the transient visual decrement that individuals report shortly after PDT treatment. Stage I is rarely seen clinically, as

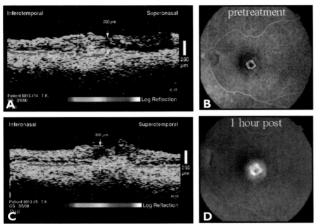

Figure 8-1. OCT (A) and fluorescein angiography (B) prior to treatment and 1 hour following PDT. The 1-hour OCT (C) and fluorescein angiography (D) studies demonstrate increased intraretinal fluid with hyperfluorescence of the CNV and treatment spot on angiography.

patients are not routinely studied during this time period. It typically resolves at the 1-week follow-up interval, and no permanent sequelae appear to result from it.

Stage II: Resolution of Subretinal Fluid With Choroidal Hypoperfusion

Approximately 1 to 2 weeks following the initial treatment, there is hypoperfusion of the CNV and choriocapillaris with a well-delineated area of hypofluorescence corresponding to the treatment spot on fluorescein angiography. The circular area of hypoperfusion is further demonstrated on indocyanine green. OCT shows resolution of subretinal fluid in the treatment zone with re-establishment of a normal foveal contour (Figure 8-2).

Choroidal hypoperfusion likely represents PDT-mediated thrombotic occlusion of the choriocapillaris.[4] The selectivity of PDT for CNV must be questioned since these findings support a more generalized choroidal perfusion deficit with secondary nonperfusion of CNV within the treated area. Hypoperfusion in the treated region may allow the retinal pigment epithelium (RPE) to pump out intra- and subretinal fluid without rapid reaccumulation from the choroid. Of interest, this is the time interval at which treated individuals report the greatest visual benefit. This logically follows given the restoration of a more normal foveal anatomy on OCT from transient elimination of intraretinal fluid collections. Stage II typically lasts up to 4 weeks until choroidal reperfusion occurs, heralding Stage III.

Stage III: Reaccumulation of Subretinal Fluid With Choroidal Reperfusion

After the fourth week of treatment, reperfusion of the CNV is present on fluorescein angiography with variable degrees of fluorescein leakage and staining. The treatment spot is less visible on angiography as the choriocapillaris is revascularized and fills rapidly. Intra- and subretinal fluid reaccumulate, and early subretinal fibrosis becomes evident on OCT between the retina and underlying RPE. This appears as a highly reflective yellow-red band between the low reflective outer retina and prominent yellow-red band of the RPE and choriocapillaris.

Stage III is subdivided into two components, depending on the ratio of retinal fluid to fibrosis. Stage IIIa has a greater retinal fluid to fibrosis ratio and represents a more active

Figure 8-2. Fluorescein angiography and OCT of Stage II lesions compared to pretreatment studies (A, B). The OCT (C) shows resolution of the intra- and subretinal fluid. There is a hypofluorescent treatment spot on angiography (D) consistent with choroidal hypoperfusion.

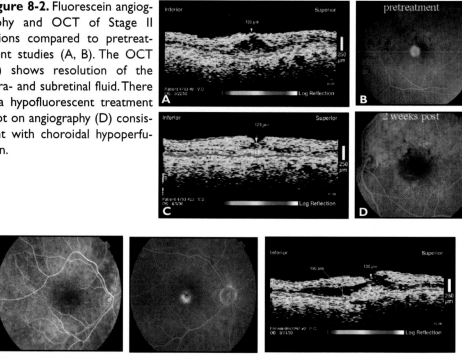

Figure 8-3. Fluorescein angiography and OCT of a Stage IIIa lesion. The OCT demonstrates recurrence of significant subretinal fluid that had previously resolved at the 1-month examination. The fluorescein angiography demonstrates an actively leaking CNV.

neovascular process. Significant leakage occurs on fluorescein angiography and prominent retinal fluid collections are identified on OCT, confirming the increased activity of the CNV (Figure 8-3). At 3 months, these patients typically require retreatment and should receive further PDT. Following retreatment, these patients repeat Stages I and II in cycle.

In contrast to Stage IIIa lesions that actively leak and require retreatment, Stage IIIb lesions are relatively inactive due to the predominance of subretinal fibrosis with minimal intra- or subretinal fluid on OCT (Figure 8-4). Stage IIIb lesions still leak on fluorescein angiography, but the fibrotic nature of the treated CNV dominates the picture and ultimately limits the central visual acuity. Treatment of lesions at this stage offers very little visual benefit, as fibrotic lesions with minimal retinal fluid fare poorly with retreatment in the authors' experience. Retreatment may lead to further contraction of the fibrotic lesion and explain the diminishing returns from multiple retreatments in patients with modest leakage. Without treatment, Stage IIIb lesions will remain stable on OCT or less often progress to Stages IV and V.

Stage IV: Subretinal Fibrosis With Persistent Retinal Fluid

The value of OCT becomes evident when analyzing Stage IV lesions. In Stage IV (Figure 8-5), replacement of the CNV with fibrosis continues and is accompanied by cystoid macular edema (CME). The CME is well documented on OCT as minimally reflective, black, circular spaces in the reflective retinal band. Angiographically, the borders of the lesion remain relatively fixed with a prominent staining component. Leakage of fluorescein persists and

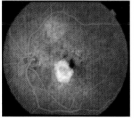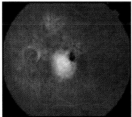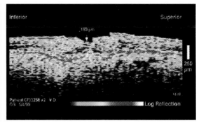

Figure 8-4. Fluorescein angiography and OCT of a Stage IIIb lesion (same patient as in Figure 8-2) 3 months after PDT. Minimal intraretinal fluid is present with a fibrotic band now present on the OCT appearing as a double red band. The fluorescein angiography shows fibrosis of the CNV, which is inactive. Staining of the lesion is present with minimal leakage.

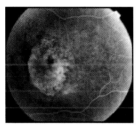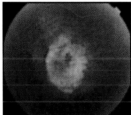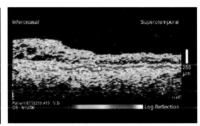

Figure 8-5. Fluorescein angiography and OCT of a Stage IV lesion. CME is prominent on the OCT and defines the type of leakage present on fluorescein angiography. The CME is off-center due to eccentric fixation (same patient as in Figures 8-2 and 8-4).

could easily be misinterpreted as leakage from an active CNV, requiring retreatment. OCT identifies the leakage on angiography as CME. At this stage, the CNV is essentially inactive. The localized leakage presumably results from dysfunctional RPE in the area of subretinal fibrosis. A Stage V lesion will naturally evolve as the CME resolves. Retreatment at this stage offers no benefit other than resolution of the macular edema.

Stage V: Subretinal Fibrosis With Retinal Atrophy

Evolution of the CNV after PDT to Stage V occurs when subretinal fibrosis organizes, retinal fluid reabsorbs, and localized retinal atrophy ensues. There is complete resolution of subretinal fluid with a subnormal central macular thickness. On OCT, the reflective band of fibrotic CNV enlarges and merges with the RPE/choriocapillaris band, obliterating the double band of fibrosis observed in Stages III and IV (Figure 8-6). The visual benefit derived from PDT is due to limitation of the final size of this stage V lesion with respect to the disciform scarring process that would have occurred without treatment.

APPLICATIONS OF THE CLASSIFICATION SYSTEM

The major prognostic indicator in predominantly classic, subfoveal CNV lesions appears to be the degree of underlying fibrosis. This often correlates to the age of the lesion and reflects the size of the lesion. Unfortunately, a lesion can exhibit characteristics that define a purely classic character, yet harbor a large element of fibrosis (Figure 8-7). CNV itself is a fibrovascular process with components of both fibrous and vascular elements in essentially

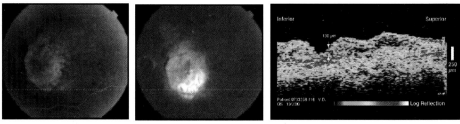

Figure 8-6. Evolution of the treated lesion from Figure 8-2. The retinal fluid has reabsorbed with localized retinal atrophy. The reflective band of fibrotic CNV has merged with the RPE/choriocapillaris band. The fluorescein angiography demonstrates prominent staining of the fibrotic lesion.

Figure 8-7. Color photo and fluorescein angiography of classic CNV with predominantly fibrotic content.

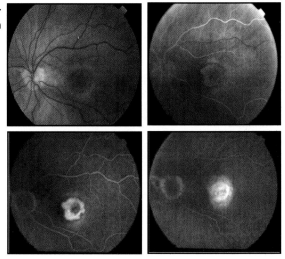

all lesions. With time, the fibrotic component will naturally predominate in the evolution toward a disciform scar. This is exactly the end-point that intervention is intended to limit. Treating a late lesion with a large fibrotic component will subject the patient to the risks of intervention without offering a significant benefit over the natural history (Figure 8-8).

It is only through careful interpretation of clinical findings and fluorescein angiography that fibrous and neovascular characteristics can be differentiated. Red-free photography is particularly useful in demonstrating whitening associated with a largely fibrotic lesion (Figure 8-9). Angiographically, the degree of staining versus leakage is very valuable in determining the fibrotic component. Finally, OCT offers an anatomic cross-section depicting the ratio of lowly reflective fluid to highly reflective fibrosis.

CASE REPORTS

Treatment of a Stage IIIa Lesion

A 72-year-old male presented with diminished visual acuity in the right eye measuring 20/60. Fluorescein angiography demonstrated a focal area of classic, subfoveal CNV with

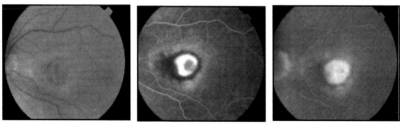

Figure 8-8. PDT of the lesion in Figure 8-7 resulting in accelerated fibrosis and corresponding decreased visual acuity. The hyperfluorescence is secondary to staining of the fibrotic lesion.

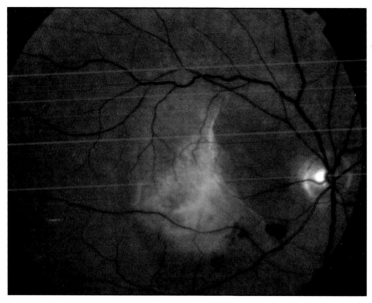

Figure 8-9. Red-free photograph of a disciform scar, which accentuates the subretinal fibrosis present.

late leakage that was corroborated on OCT (Figures 8-10 and 8-11). PDT with verteporfin was performed by standard protocol. Four weeks following treatment, the visual acuity improved to 20/50. A Stage II lesion was identified on OCT with reduction in subretinal fluid and a near-normal foveal contour (Figure 8-12). There was delayed filling with minimal late leakage of fluorescein from the lesion on angiography (Figure 8-13). Three months after PDT, the visual acuity diminished to 20/100. Clinical examination, fluorescein angiography, and OCT revealed increased subretinal fluid consistent with a Stage IIIa lesion (Figures 8-14 and 8-15), qualifying for retreatment. Following retreatment, the visual acuity improved to 20/50 with minimal leakage of the lesion on fluorescein angiography, and the OCT staging system has recycled and returned to a Stage II lesion (Figures 8-16 and 8-17). Three months following retreatment, the visual acuity remained 20/60 without sub- or intraretinal fluid on OCT. Six months following retreatment, the visual acuity remained stable at 20/60 and a Stage IIIb lesion was identified on OCT with minimal staining on fluorescein angiography. The patient continues to be observed.

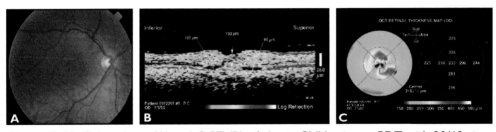

Figure 8-10. Color photo (A) and OCT (B) of classic CNV prior to PDT with 20/60 visual acuity. The CNV is visible as a highly reflective, red-yellow band in the subretinal space above the RPE/choriocapillaris layer. Mild subretinal fluid surrounds the CNV in the subfoveal space and is represented by the absence of signal. The topographic map (C) shows increased macular thickness in the foveal and parafoveal regions.

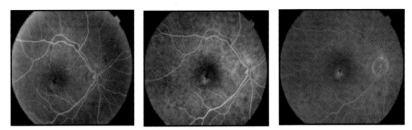

Figure 8-11. Fluorescein angiography corresponding to the OCT in Figure 8-10 demonstrating a small, classic CNV with late leakage. PDT was performed.

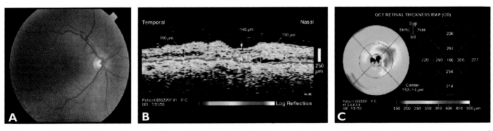

Figure 8-12. Color photo (A) and OCT (B, C) 1 month after PDT showing restoration of foveal anatomy with reduced macular thickness. The OCT represents a Stage II lesion. Mild subretinal fluid persisted and the visual acuity improved to 20/50.

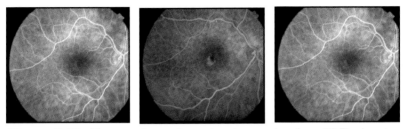

Figure 8-13. Fluorescein angiography 1 month after PDT showing decreased leakage of the CNV with mild hypofluorescence in the treatment zone.

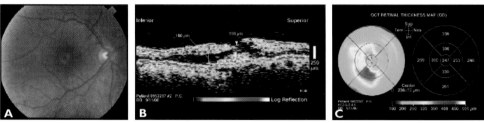

Figure 8-14. Color photo (A) and OCT (B, C) 3 months after PDT with reaccumulation of subretinal fluid and increased macular thickening. Subretinal fluid is prominent as a nonreflective zone under the retinal reflection. Mild subretinal fibrosis is present in the fovea as a thickened, highly reflective, yellow-red band. A Stage IIIa lesion is present, as there is greater subretinal fluid to fibrosis ratio. The vision decreased to 20/100.

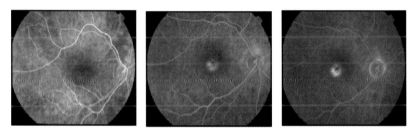

Figure 8-15. The fluorescein angiogram at 3 months showing increased leakage from the subfoveal CNV that corresponds with the reaccumulation of subretinal fluid on OCT. Based on the increased subretinal fluid (Stage IIIa lesion) and decreased visual acuity, retreatment with PDT was performed.

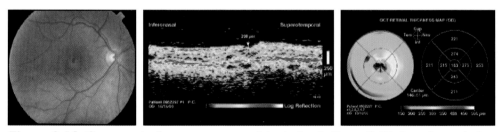

Figure 8-16. One month after retreatment of the lesion in Figure 8-15, there is resolution of subretinal fluid and macular thickening (Stage II lesion) with improvement of the visual acuity to 20/50. This demonstrates how retreatment of a Stage IIIa lesion restarts the classification cycle.

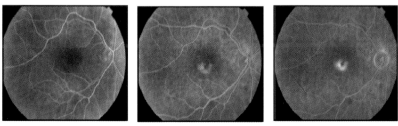

Figure 8-17. Fluorescein angiography 1 month after retreatment shows early hypofluorescence in the area of the treatment spot with leakage in the later frames. Despite the fluorescein leakage, the patient was observed as the OCT reveals a Stage II lesion with minimal intraretinal fluid.

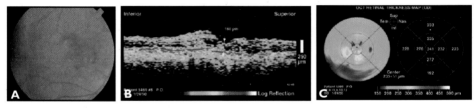

Figure 8-18. Color photo (A) and OCT (B, C) of subfoveal CNV 9 months after initial PDT and two retreatments. On OCT, the subretinal fibrosis is prominent with minimal subretinal fluid representing a Stage IIIb lesion. The visual acuity is 20/200.

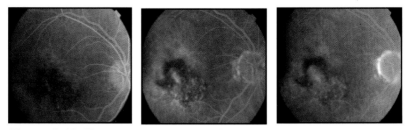

Figure 8-19. Fluorescein angiography demonstrating progressive staining of a predominantly fibrotic lesion with minimal late leakage corresponding to the Stage IIIb OCT lesion. No further PDT was performed and the patient was observed.

Observation of a Stage IIIb Lesion With Subsequent Treatment of a Stage IV Lesion

A 78-year-old female with predominantly classic CNV and 20/400 visual acuity was treated with PDT. Following treatment, the visual acuity remained stable with a Stage IIIb lesion on OCT with diminished leakage on fluorescein angiography 3 months following treatment (Figures 8-18 and 8-19). Given the early subretinal fibrosis and diminished subretinal fluid, the patient was observed. Six months after treatment, the visual acuity remained 20/200 with increased subretinal fluid on clinical examination. CME was identified on OCT (Figure 8-20). Fluorescein angiography (Figure 8-21) demonstrated increased leakage, which was interpreted as recurrent CNV. PDT was repeated based on the angiographic appearance. Three months after the second treatment, the visual acuity measured 20/400 and the OCT demonstrated a Stage V lesion with retinal atrophy and fibrosis (Figures 8-22 and 8-23).

In retrospect, observation of the Stage IIIb lesion was likely a sound clinical decision. Fluorescein interpretation of CME can be deceptive as leakage into the cystoid spaces as identified in a Stage IV OCT can mimic the angiographic appearance of an active CNV. OCT aids in differentiating between fluorescein leakage from active CNV in Stage IIIa lesions and CME in Stage IV lesions with fibrotic CNV. This case demonstrates how treatment of a Stage IV lesion leads to retinal atrophy and accelerates progression to a Stage V lesion.

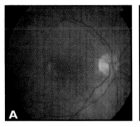 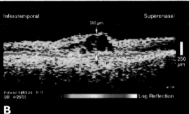 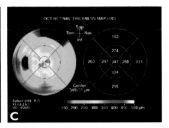

Figure 8-20. Color photo (A) and OCT (B, C) 3 months after the studies were performed in Figures 8-18 and 8-19. CME has naturally evolved with minimal subretinal fibrosis creating a Stage IV lesion. The vision is 20/400. The initial treatment was performed 12 months prior to these photos, with the last retreatment 6 months prior to these studies.

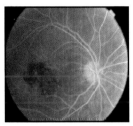 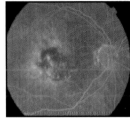 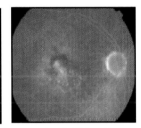

Figure 8-21. Fluorescein angiography corresponding to the OCT in Figure 8-20 showing continued staining of a fibrotic CNV with late leakage confirmed to be CME on OCT. Note that this lesion does not significantly differ from Figure 8-19 angiographically despite significant CME.

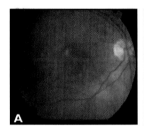 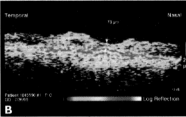 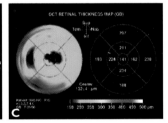

Figure 8-22. Color photo (A) and OCT (B, C) 9 months following the last retreatment showing natural progression to a limited disciform scar (Stage V). Note the large fibrotic subretinal complex, absence of retinal fluid, thinning, and atrophy of the overlying neurosensory retina. The visual acuity remains 20/400.

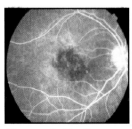 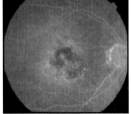 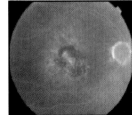

Figure 8-23. Fluorescein angiography of the CNV in Figure 8-22 shows persistent staining of a fibrotic CNV. Note the similar appearance to Figures 8-19 and 8-21 angiographically despite dramatic changes in retinal fluid content as observed on OCT.

Figure 8-24. OCT of the left eye at baseline (A) and 3 months later (B) when the patient presented with diminished visual acuity. The pretreatment OCT (B) identifies mild intraretinal fluid.

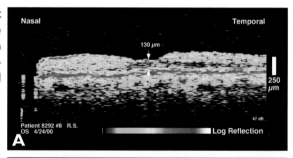

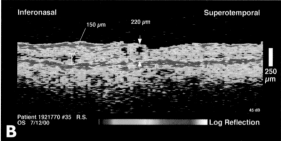

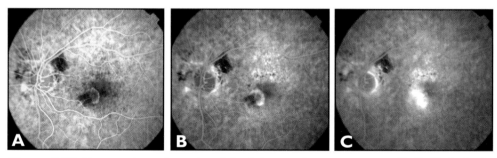

Figure 8-25. Fluorescein angiography of the left eye prior to treatment (A, B, C). A classic subfoveal CNV with late leakage is identified. The visual acuity measures 20/30.

Treatment of Stage II/IIIb Lesions

An 85-year-old female with AMD and a disciform scar in her right eye presented with diminished visual acuity measuring 20/30 in the left eye. OCT demonstrated mild subretinal fluid compared to her normal OCT performed 3 months earlier (Figure 8-24). A classic, subfoveal CNV was identified on fluorescein angiography with late leakage (Figure 8-25). PDT was performed with verteporfin. One month following treatment, the patient complained of decreased visual acuity measuring 20/50. On angiography the margins of the lesion were blunted but leaked later in the study. Reduction of intraretinal fluid was present on OCT, consistent with a Stage II/IIIb lesion (Figure 8-26). Given the persistent leakage and decreased visual acuity, the lesion was retreated with verteporfin at 1 month. Two weeks following retreatment, the patient was re-examined with a reduction in vision to 20/100 without significant change in her OCT. The OCT was interpreted as a Stage II lesion. On fluorescein angiography, there was persistent blunting of the margins of the lesion with evidence of late staining. Minimal leakage of fluorescein dye was evident (Figure 8-27). Six weeks following retreatment, the visual acuity declined to 20/400 with a Stage V lesion.

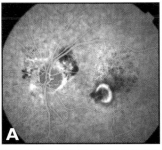
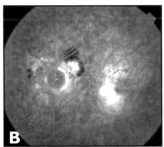
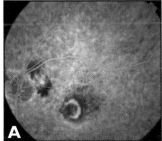
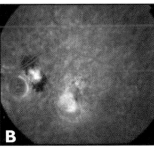
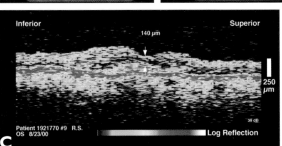

Figure 8-26. Fluorescein angiography (A, B) of the left eye 1 month after PDT with verteporfin. The CNV is still visible angiographically with blunting of the margins (A) and late leakage (B). A Stage II lesion is revealed on OCT with minimal intraretinal fluid and a normal appearing fovea contour (C). The visual acuity measures 20/50.

Figure 8-27. Two weeks following retreatment, the visual acuity declined to 20/100. Fluorescein angiography reveals persistent blunting of the margins of the lesion (A) with late staining (B). Minimal leakage of fluorescein dye is visible. OCT reveals a Stage II lesion (C).

Retinal atrophy with subretinal fibrosis is identified on OCT. Angiography revealed an inactive lesion with staining of fibrosis (Figure 8-28).

This case demonstrates the value of OCT in regard to retreatment of CNV using PDT. Subretinal fluid appears to directly correlate with the activity of the CNV. Lesions with more prominent sub- and intraretinal fluid characteristics, as seen in Stage IIIa lesions, represent more active CNV. Lesions that are clinically inactive on angiography and OCT do not appear to benefit from further treatment. In this situation, the patient was retreated with a Stage II/IIIb lesion that demonstrated minimal intra- and subretinal fluid. Retreatment induced a more aggressive response to the photosensitizing agent and acceler-

Figure 8-28. Six weeks following retreatment, the red-free photograph highlights the fibrosis (A). Fluorescein angiography (B, C, D) and OCT (E) reveal an inactive lesion with fibrosis and retinal atrophy.

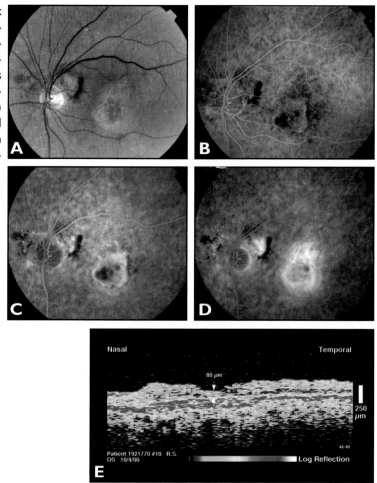

ated the involutional process of the CNV. The lesion rapidly progressed from a Stage II lesion following retreatment to a Stage V lesion with retinal atrophy and subretinal fibrosis.

Currently, retreatment of CNV with PDT is advocated at the 3-month visit if angiographically warranted.[1] The TAP Study Group did not evaluate retreatment at earlier intervals. In some situations this may be warranted, especially if significant subretinal fluid and leakage from the CNV is present, as is seen in Stage IIIa lesions. In the above case report, the lack of subretinal fluid on OCT identified the inactivity of the lesion. Observation was likely warranted in this clinical situation.

SUMMARY

A five-stage PDT classification system appears useful in understanding the events that follow treatment with this technique. Stage I represents an acute, transient inflammatory response to the photodynamic process. Resolution is heralded by Stage II, in which the choriocapillaris is temporarily hypoperfused; OCT shows resolution of retinal fluid with establishment of a more normal foveal contour. Visual benefit appears greatest at this stage.

However, Stage III is inevitable as the choriocapillaris and CNV are reperfused. The degree of fluid and fibrosis determine whether a lesion will be classified as Stage IIIa or IIIb. Stage III usually is evident at the 3-month follow-up interval, at which time a decision for retreatment is required. Stage IIIa lesions have a relatively low degree of fibrosis with a more prominent fluid component. These lesions typically benefit from retreatment and start the classification cycle over when treated again. Stage IIIb lesions, however, exhibit higher levels of fibrosis than fluid and do not respond well to retreatment. Vision is limited by the fibrotic component, and the lesions either remain stable at IIIb or less commonly progress to Stage IV and V. In Stage IV, CME persists over fibrotic CNV and dysfunctional RPE. These lesions are relatively stable, as the CNV is essentially inactive and the retina is responding to a localized subretinal fibrosis. The end stage is Stage V, in which fluid is replaced by a fibrotic scar with overlying retinal atrophy. The size of the final lesion determines visual outcome. PDT is effective in limiting the proportion of this component to reduce moderate visual loss.

As far as implications for treatment and retreatment, cases should be selected that have a vascular component that is greater than the fibrotic component. The degree of fibrosis can be evaluated clinically and is reflected by the appearance, age, and size of the lesion. It appears that smaller, more acute lesions fare better with PDT due to creation of a smaller ultimate scotoma after fibrosis of the neovascular complex. Caution must be exercised when treating lesions with a larger fibrotic component, as these lesions tend to scar rapidly and are prone to hemorrhage.

Retreatment can be limited by deferring further treatment once Stage IIIb or later is reached. At these later stages, the lesion has been essentially inactivated and further treatment will only accelerate ultimate fibrosis. Subretinal fibrosis results in overlying retinal atrophy and local visual dysfunction. Just as conventional laser induces an immediate scotoma through destruction of photoreceptors, PDT causes a delayed scotoma due to progressive retinal atrophy over a fibrosed choroidal neovascular complex.

While the OCT classification system may ultimately limit the number of retreatments, this staging system has been compiled in a retrospective review of the authors' cases and has not been tested in a prospective fashion. The decision to treat subfoveal CNV with PDT cannot be based on OCT alone. OCT is a tool that adds another dimension to fluorescein angiography by providing a cross-sectional view of the retina. While OCT may ultimately be used to modify the approach to retreatment, the TAP study still remains the standard by which retreatment should be based, as it has been proven in a randomized, double-blind study.

REFERENCES

1. Treatment of Age-Related Macular Degeneration with Photodynamic Therapy Study Group. Photodynamic therapy of subfoveal choroidal neovascularization in age-related macular degeneration with verteporfin. *Arch Ophthalmol*. 1999;117:1329-1345.

2. Roberts WG, Hasan T. Role of neovasculature permeability on the tumor retention of photodynamic agents. *Cancer Res*. 1992;52:924-930.

3. Brown SG, Tralau PD, Smith D. Photodynamic therapy with porphyrin and phthalocyanines sensitization: quantitative studies in normal rat liver. *Br J Cancer*. 1986;54:43-52.

4. Henderson BW, Dougherty TJ. How does photodynamic therapy work? *Photochem Photobiol*. 1992;55:145-157.

5. Moan J, Peng, Q, Evensen JF, et al. Photosensitizing efficiencies, tumor and cellular uptake of different photosensitizing drugs relevant for photodynamic therapy of cancer. *Photochem Photobiol*. 1987;46:713-721.

6. Rosenthal I. Phthalocyanines as photosensitizers. *Photochem Photobiol.* 1991;53:859-870.

7. Obana A, Gohto Y, Kanai M, et al. Selective photodynamic effects of the new photosensitizer ATX-S10(Na) on choroidal neovascularization in monkeys. *Arch Ophthalmol.* 2000;118:650-658.

8. Roberts WG, Smith M, McCullough JL, Berns MW. Skin photosensitivity and photodestruction of several potential photodynamic sensitizers. *Photochem Photobiol.* 1989;49:431-438.

CHAPTER NINE

OPHTHALMIC COMPLICATIONS OF PHOTODYNAMIC THERAPY FOR CHOROIDAL NEOVASCULARIZATION

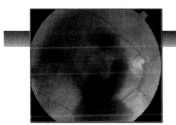 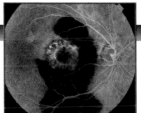 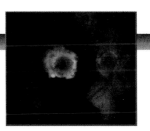

CHAPTER SECTIONS

Photodynamic therapy (PDT) is generally a safe procedure when performed in accordance with accepted treatment guidelines.[1] Proper case selection will allow the most efficacious treatment of patients without subjecting poor candidates to the potential risks of therapy. Although ophthalmic complications are not commonly seen with PDT, negative outcomes can be devastating in the intended patient population. Many prospective PDT candidates have poor visual function at baseline and a large percentage are functionally monocular. This chapter will review some of the complications and negative outcomes of PDT. Causative patterns will be evaluated along with rationales for the avoidance of such poor outcomes.

SUBRETINAL HEMORRHAGE

Treatment of more chronic lesions may be associated with the development of subretinal hemorrhage. Hemorrhage has traditionally been attributed to new or recurrent choroidal neovascularization (CNV). However, it appears that PDT of lesions with large fibrotic components often results in hemorrhage at the edge of the neovascular complex. This may be due to contraction of the fibrosing lesion with traction on the feeding vessels. PDT appears to enhance this process by accelerating fibrosis. In the phases 1 and 2 study of verteporfin,[1] 8.6% of treated patients experienced increased subretinal hemorrhage and 3.1% experienced new subretinal hemorrhage. In the authors' experience, treatment of more acute lesions with PDT rarely results in subretinal hemorrhage.

Case Report: Subretinal Hemorrhage After Treatment of Chronic Choroidal Neovascularization

A 67-year-old female presented with diminished visual acuity measuring 20/60 and a relatively small, choroidal neovascular membrane in the left eye. The lesion was 100% classic and subfoveal (Figure 9-1), qualifying the patient for treatment with PDT, which was performed without complication. Three months later, she returned with progressive visual decline to 20/200. Fluorescein angiography showed staining of subretinal fibrosis in the area of previously active CNV with new hemorrhage along the superotemporal border. Late frames did show evidence of minimal persistent leakage (Figure 9-2). Re-evaluation of the presenting angiogram showed a large underlying fibrotic component resulting in mild late leakage. Given our current experience with PDT, this patient would likely have been best observed at the presenting stage. Final vision was 20/400 6 months post-treatment.

Case Report: Large Subretinal Hemorrhage After Photodynamic Therapy of Chronic Choroidal Neovascularization

A 79-year-old male presented with progressive visual loss and distortion in the right eye. Fluorescein angiography was performed and showed a subfoveal, classic choroidal neovascular membrane (Figure 9-3). Vision measured 20/200. The patient qualified for PDT and was treated without complication. Three months later, the patient reported no improvement in his visual status. Clinical examination revealed a large submacular hemorrhage surrounding the previous neovascular complex (Figure 9-4). Fluorescein angiography showed minimal leakage from this largely fibrotic lesion with blockage by the subretinal hemorrhage. Remarkably, vision remained 20/200 at this interval.

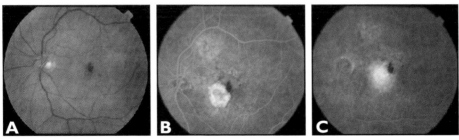

Figure 9-1. A 67-year-old female with a classic, subfoveal CNV and 20/60 visual acuity was treated with photodynamic therapy (A). Closer inspection of the angiogram demonstrates signs of chronicity, despite late leakage (C). The boarders of the lesion are fixed (B) and the body of the lesion stains, suggesting prominent fibrosis (B, C).

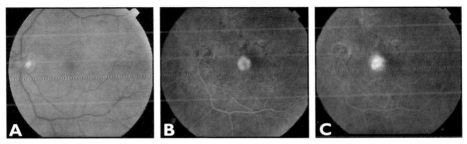

Figure 9-2. Three months after PDT of the lesion in Figure 9-1. Visual acuity has declined to 20/200. Subretinal fibrosis is evident both on the color photo (A) and the angiogram with prominent staining (B, C).

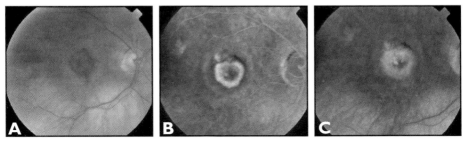

Figure 9-3. A classic, subfoveal CNV in a 79-year-old male referred for treatment by PDT. While the lesion demonstrates late leakage (A), the lesion margins are quite blunted with staining (B, C). Visual acuity measured 20/200 and PDT was performed.

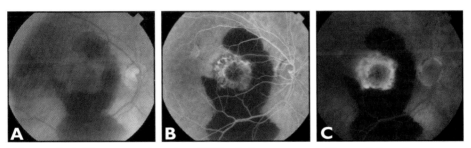

Figure 9-4. Three months after PDT of the patient in Figure 9-3, color photos demonstrate significant subretinal hemorrhage (A). There is persistent leakage with staining of the lesion (B, C).

EXUBERANT SUBRETINAL FIBROSIS

It appears that the benefit of PDT derives from the cessation of leakage from active CNV through subretinal fibrosis. The final scotoma is relatively smaller compared to disciform scarring from the natural evolution of the neovascular process. However, treatment of lesions with a large fibrotic component at baseline appears to increase the risk of exuberant subretinal fibrosis with subsequent significant visual loss. In the phases 1 and 2 study of verteporfin,[1] 8.6% of treated patients showed increased subretinal fibrosis associated with CNV. Multiple etiologies appear plausible to explain this phenomenon, and all may play a role in causing ultimate loss of vision. The fibrotic component may progressively stain with photosensitizer (analogous to fluorescein staining), resulting in a higher concentration of agent in the area of CNV. This may result in an effective "overdosage" in these cases. The retina is often attenuated over chronic neovascular tissue and may be more susceptible to damage after photoactivation. Finally, choroidal blood flow is likely altered in the areas of fibrosing CNV, altering the pharmacokinetics of photosensitizer accumulation and clearance.

Case Report: Treatment of Chronic Lesion

A 74-year-old female presented with progressive visual loss in the right eye. Fluorescein angiography showed 100% classic, subfoveal CNV measuring 2700 microns in the greatest linear dimension (Figure 9-5). Visual acuity measured 20/160 and PDT was performed. Three months later, the patient returned with progressive visual loss to 20/400. Fluorescein angiography showed subretinal fibrosis in the area of prior active CNV with a surrounding neurosensory detachment corresponding to the treatment spot (Figure 9-6). Optical coherence tomography (OCT) confirmed this localized detachment of the neurosensory retina. Re-evaluation of the presenting angiogram shows minimal late leakage from a largely fibrotic classic neovascular lesion. Further follow-up showed progressive visual loss to the counting fingers level. The natural history would likely compare favorably with the treatment outcome, but with a slower progression.

Case Report: Treatment of Chronic Lesion

A 76-year-old male presented with diminished acuity and metamorphopsia in the right eye. Vision measured 20/160. Fluorescein angiography showed subfoveal classic CNV that qualified for treatment with PDT (Figure 9-7). At 3 months, vision decreased to 20/400 and leakage persisted. Retreatment was performed. Over the next several months, vision continued to deteriorate to the counting fingers level. Subretinal fibrosis progressed with hemorrhage at the edge of the neovascular complex (Figure 9-8). Both fibrosis and hemorrhage are shown to result from treatment of a chronic neovascular lesion, despite its classic character.

NEUROSENSORY RETINAL DETACHMENT

Neurosensory retinal detachment is a complication of PDT that was elucidated in prior studies of PDT with various photosensitizers.[2,3] This manifests as a circumscribed serous elevation of the retina in the area of the treatment spot. The clinical picture may resemble central serous chorioretinopathy. The etiology is unclear but may represent damage to the retinal pigment epithelium (RPE) with inability to pump out accumulated subretinal fluid.

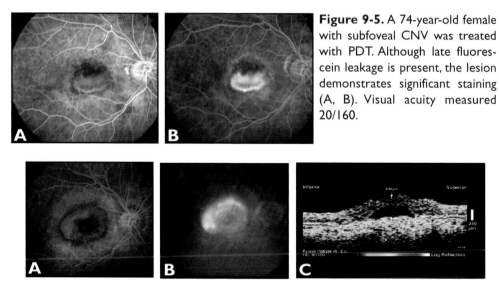

Figure 9-5. A 74-year-old female with subfoveal CNV was treated with PDT. Although late fluorescein leakage is present, the lesion demonstrates significant staining (A, B). Visual acuity measured 20/160.

Figure 9-6. Three months after PDT of the patient in Figure 9-5, visual acuity measured 20/400. Progressive staining is visible on angiography (A, B) with leakage into the subretinal space, as demonstrated by the neurosensory detachment on OCT (C). Visual acuity eventually declined to counting fingers.

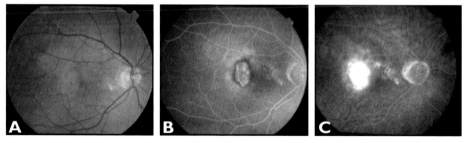

Figure 9-7. A 76-year-old male with subfoveal CNV was treated with PDT. Color photo (A) shows evidence of fibrosis, which is identified by staining on angiography (B, C). Given the late leakage, PDT was performed.

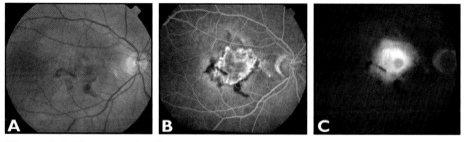

Figure 9-8. Three months after treatment, there is evidence of increased fibrosis with surrounding subretinal hemorrhage (A). The lesion has enlarged on angiography (B) with staining (C). Vision has declined from 20/160 to 20/400 after treatment.

Figure 9-9. A classic subfoveal CNV (A, B) with 20/200 visual acuity was treated with PDT.

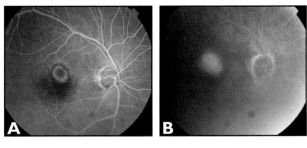

Figure 9-10. One month following treatment of the CNV in Figure 9-9, the lesion remains stable. There is mild hyperfluorescence delineating the treatment zone surrounding the lesion (A, B).

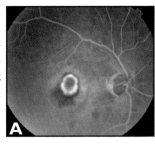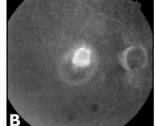

Figure 9-11. Three months after treatment the vision remained stable at 20/200. There is angiographic evidence of a neurosensory detachment (A, B), which was confirmed on OCT.

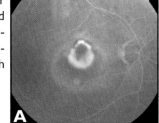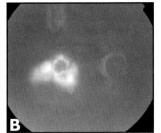

Case Report: Neurosensory Retinal Detachment

An 82-year-old male presented with progressive visual loss associated with classic, subfoveal CNV. Vision measured 20/200 and fluorescein angiography confirmed the presence of a qualifying lesion for PDT (Figure 9-9). At 1 month, the lesion began to show angiographic evidence of regression. There was a faint hyperfluorescent rim corresponding to the treatment spot (Figure 9-10). At 3 months, the lesion did not change significantly. There was, however, a large subretinal fluid collection in the distribution of the treatment spot (Figure 9-11). This was confirmed by OCT. Fluorescein angiography showed leakage in the subretinal space that appeared distinct from the neovascular process. Vision did remain 20/200 despite the presence of a neurosensory retinal detachment involving the fovea. The patient's age may have played a role in the development of this complication, as this trend has been noticed in affected patients. Further study is necessary to confirm a relationship.

MACULAR INFARCTION

Retinal capillary nonperfusion has been reported after PDT. A higher incidence was demonstrated in phase 1 and 2 trials[4] where the light dose, or fluence, was increased to 150 J/cm^2 in a subset of patients. In this trial, 2.3% of treated subjects experienced branch reti-

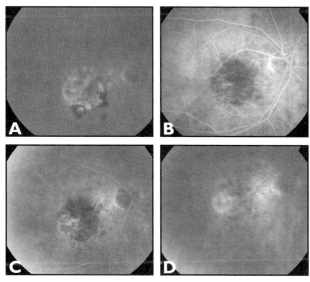

Figure 9-12. The pretreatment angiogram in this 78-year-old female demonstrates an occult subfoveal CNV treated with verteporfin (A). Visual acuity measured 20/400. Four months after treatment, a circular area of delayed choroidal hypoperfusion in the treatment zone persisted in early, middle, and late frames of the angiogram (B, C, D). Visual acuity remains 20/400.

nal arteriolar or venular nonperfusion. Overdosage has also been associated with macular infarction due to occlusion of large retinal vessels. This argues against selectivity of PDT for choroidal neovascular tissue. Fortunately, macular infarction and capillary nonperfusion are not frequently encountered with proper dosing and laser parameters. This complication has not been experienced at our treatment center.

The authors have experienced two cases of persistent choroidal hypoperfusion following PDT using verteporfin. While hypoperfused treatment spots are common on follow-up angiography within 1 month of treatment, this angiographic finding is usually transient as the choroid reperfuses. In the two cases identified by the authors, the hypoperfused treatment spot has been identified as much as 4 months after a single treatment. This appears to occur in older individuals and may be related to vascular disease affecting the choroidal vessels.

Case Report: Persistent Choroidal Hypoperfusion After PDT

A 78-year-old female with an occult CNV, identified in 1999, presented after a 2-year absence with a decline in visual acuity from 20/80 to 20/400. Fluorescein angiography revealed enlargement of the occult, subfoveal CNV (Figure 9-12 [A]). Her medical history was significant for systemic lupus erythematosus, hypertension, and a previous stroke. Medications included hydroxychloroquine 200 mg daily, three antihypertensive medications, and coumadin. Given the growth of her occult lesion with a decline in visual acuity, PDT with verteporfin was performed. The patient returned 4 months later with the visual acuity unchanged at 20/400. Angiography demonstrated a circular, hypoperfused treatment spot that persisted throughout the fluorescein angiogram (Figure 9-12 [B, C, D]). The patient noted no significant change in vision and remained asymptomatic despite the finding. She continues to be followed.

REFERENCES

1. Treatment of Age-Related Macular Degeneration with Photodynamic Therapy Study Group. Photodynamic therapy of subfoveal choroidal neovascularization in age-related macular degeneration with verteporfin. *Arch Ophthalmol.* 1999;117:1329-1345.

2. Kliman GH, Puliafito CA, Stern D, et al. Phthalocyanine photodynamic therapy: new strategy for closure of choroidal neovascularization. *Lasers Surg Med.* 1994;15:2-10.

3. Peyman G, Moshfeghi DM, Moshfeghi A, et al. Photodynamic therapy for choriocapillaris using tin ethyl etiopurpin (SnET2). *Ophthalmic Surg Lasers.* 1997;28:409-417.

4. Miller JW, Schmidt-Erfurth U, Sickenberg M, et al. Photodynamic therapy with verteporfin for choroidal neovascularization caused by age-related macular degeneration: results of a single treatment in a phase 1 and 2 study. *Arch Ophthalmol.* 1999;117:1161-1173.

CHAPTER TEN

ALTERNATIVE APPLICATIONS OF PHOTODYNAMIC THERAPY

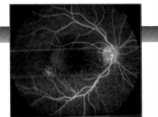 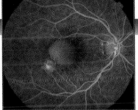 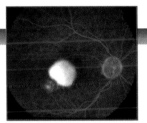

CHAPTER SECTIONS

- ❖ Serous Pigment Epithelial Detachment
- ❖ Occult Choroidal Neovascularization
- ❖ Pattern Dystrophy
- ❖ Indocyanine Green Hot Spots
- ❖ Polypoidal Choroidal Vasculopathy
- ❖ Angioid Streaks
- ❖ Idiopathic CNV
- ❖ Conclusion

While photodynamic therapy (PDT) has proven efficacious in the treatment of predominantly classic, subfoveal choroidal neovascularization (CNV) from age-related macular degeneration (AMD),[1,2] its application toward other choroidal vascular abnormalities has not been established. Using case examples, this chapter explores alternative applications of PDT for the treatment of polypoidal choroidal vasculopathy (PCV), occult CNV, serous pigment epithelial detachment (PED), CNV associated with pattern dystrophy, and focal spots delineated on indocyanine green angiography. While these are considered "off-label" uses, PDT was offered as an option for patients who either failed to qualify or refused other non-PDT forms of treatment. Examples of CNV associated with angioid streaks and idiopathic CNV are also reported. The authors of this text do not advocate the widespread use of PDT in the clinical examples given. Other than occult CNV, these alternate uses of PDT have not been proven effective. These examples are included for the benefit of the reader only.

SEROUS PIGMENT EPITHELIAL DETACHMENT

A 68-year-old female with AMD presented with a 2-month history of diminished visual acuity in the right eye. Visual acuity measured 20/200 OD with a serous PED on biomicroscopy. A circular, well-defined lesion that uniformly filled with early hyperfluorescence adjacent to a punctate area of retinal hyperfluorescence was present on fluorescein angiography. The area corresponding to the serous PED was hypofluorescent on indocyanine green angiography. Optical coherence tomography (OCT) demonstrated a 590-micron serous cavity with a normal appearing retina and retinal pigment epithelial (RPE) cell layer (Figure 10-1). PDT with verteporfin was administered by standard protocol. Examination 2 days following treatment revealed improved visual acuity to 20/40 OD with a diminished serous PED (Figure 10-2). One week following treatment, the visual acuity improved to 20/30 with further reduction in the serous PED (Figure 10-3). Four months following treatment, the corrected visual acuity measured 20/25 despite an enlargement of the serous cavity to 490 microns measured on OCT. Retreatment with PDT was performed twice over the next 4 months with fluctuations in the size of the serous PED. Eight months following the initial treatment the visual acuity measured 20/50 with persistence of the serous PED (Figure 10-4).

Serous PED is a round or oval, dome-shaped elevation of intact neurosensory retina and RPE overlying sub-RPE fluid. Fluorescein angiography demonstrates early hyperfluorescence with pooling of fluorescein dye that continues to hyperfluoresce after the recirculation phase. The serous PED is hypofluorescent on indocyanine green angiography. Poliner et al[3] evaluated the natural history of serous PEDs that occurred within a 2500-micron radius from the foveal avascular zone. With a mean follow-up of over 24 months, patients with serous PEDs were more likely to have a visual acuity measuring 20/20 to 20/50 than other forms of PED (hemorrhagic or turbid PEDs). At 36 months, slightly greater than 50% of the patients had a visual acuity of 20/200 or better. Eyes that progressed to CNV tended to be older than 65 years of age, have a larger detachment (1000 microns or greater), subretinal fluid present, and disciform scar in the fellow eye. At 3 years, 49% of eyes with serous PED developed CNV.

Meredith et al[4] evaluated the natural history of serous PED over a mean follow-up of 22 months. Risk factors for the development of CNV mirrored those observed by Poliner and associates. These included age greater than 56 years, serous detachments larger than 1 disk diameter, and the presence of subretinal fluid. Spontaneous resolution of the detachment resulted in mild atrophy of the RPE most pronounced on fluorescein angiography. Visual

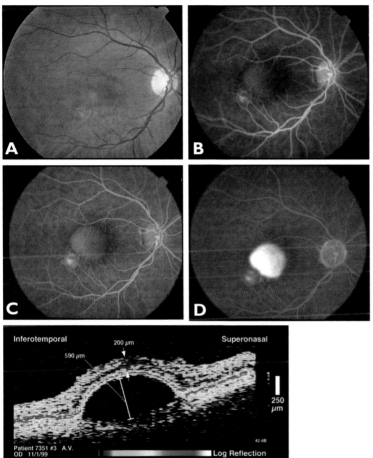

Figure 10-1. Color photo (A) and fluorescein angiography (B, C, D) with uniform hyperfluorescence in a circular pattern consistent with a serous PED in the right eye. OCT measures the PED cavity at 590 microns with an intact overlying retina and RPE layer (E). The visual acuity is 20/200 OD.

outcome was age related. In patients younger than 55 years, 81.8% of eyes had a visual acuity of 20/80 or better at the beginning of the study, while 90.9% of eyes achieved this level at the end of the study. In older patients, 87.1% started the study 20/80 or better, while only 53.8% reached this level at the conclusion of follow-up.

In 64 eyes with serous PED, Casswell et al[5] recognized separate outcomes of untreated lesions. Thirty percent developed CNV, spontaneous flattening occurred in 17%, and tears of the RPE in 10%. Flattening of the PED was associated with RPE atrophy and diminished visual acuity. Persistence of the PED was the only lesion classification that maintained consistently good vision.

Treatment of serous PEDs has consisted of laser photocoagulation to the lesion. In 1974, Bird[6] published the treatment results of 24 serous PEDs. Laser was applied in a continuous linear fashion around the base of the lesion with grid laser densely placed over the body of the PED while avoiding the fovea. Of the 24 lesions, 21 remained flat after treatment. The detachment persisted in two, and one patient developed CNV 6 months after retinal flattening. Visual acuity improved in 15 and remained unchanged in eight eyes after treatment. The high rate of successful anatomic flattening and visual recovery prompted a recommendation that serous PEDs without evidence of CNV should be treated until flat.

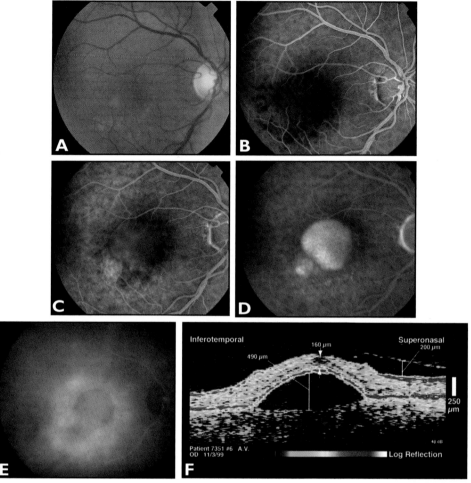

Figure 10-2. Two days following treatment, the visual acuity improved to 20/40 OD (A). There is sluggish filling of the serous PED with fluorescein compared to the pretreatment fluorescein angiography (B, C, D). The fluorescein angiography at 31.5 seconds delineates the hypoperfused treatment spot (B) with partial filling of the PED at 1 minute (C). The PED cavity is filled at 5 minutes (D). The hypofluorescent area on indocyanine green angiography, representing the PED, is now surrounded by a rim of hyperfluorescence consistent with the circular treatment spot (E). This hyperfluorescent rim is likely secondary to inflammation induced from activation of the photosensitizing agent. OCT shows a decrease in the cavity of the serous PED to 490 microns (F).

Subsequent evaluation of laser photocoagulation of serous PEDs demonstrated no benefit. Braunstein and Gass[7] in 1979 retrospectively reviewed 24 untreated with 21 treated eyes with serous PEDs associated with AMD. The authors found no conclusive evidence that photocoagulation of the PED altered the natural history. The Moorfields Macular Study Group[8] further evaluated argon laser photocoagulation of serous PEDs in a prospective, randomized, controlled trial. Treated eyes experienced a significant deterioration in visual acuity within 3 months of treatment compared with untreated eyes, prompting the Data

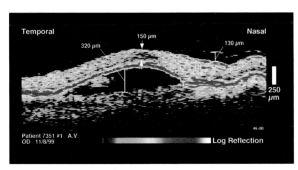

Figure 10-3. OCT 1 week following treatment demonstrating a decrease in the cavity size of the serous PED to 320 microns. The visual acuity improved to 20/30 OD.

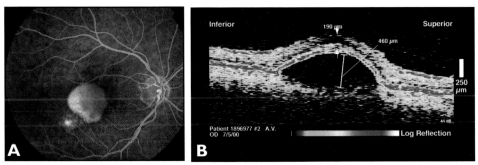

Figure 10-4. Eight months following treatment, the visual acuity measures 20/50. The fluorescein angiography (A) and OCT (B) show a persistent PED.

Monitoring Committee to terminate recruitment of patients. At 18 months, 73% of treatment eyes and 41% of untreated eyes experienced a 2-line reduction in visual acuity. The trial concluded that photocoagulation of serous PEDs provided no visual benefit over observation. Barondes et al evaluated the 4-year follow-up results of the remaining 15 treated and 19 untreated eyes from the Moorfields Macular Study Group.[9] While visual acuity remained stable in the treatment group, the untreated eyes followed the natural history of disease with gradual loss of vision. The treated group lost 3.33 lines of visual acuity compared with 3.37 lines lost in the control eyes at 4 years. Not until after year 2 did the control group show a decline in visual acuity similar to the treatment arm, demonstrating that treatment accelerated visual loss. Geographic atrophy was more common in the laser-treated eyes, but the occurrence of CNV and tears of the RPE were equal in the two groups. Persistence of the serous detachment occurred only in the untreated group. As identified in a previous study,[5] eyes with persistent PED had the best visual outcome losing only 1 line of acuity.

PDT temporarily decreases the sub-RPE fluid in a serous PED. The mechanism by which this occurs is unknown but appears to be related to temporary choroidal and choriocapillaris hypoperfusion induced in the treatment area. This is a reproducible finding on fluorescein and indocyanine green angiography following PDT with verteporfin in all cases. Reperfusion of the treatment area occurs within 4 weeks after PDT and corresponds with reaccumulation of the serous component of the PED. Another hypothesis explaining the failure of PDT treatment of serous PEDs is that the absorptive property of the serous fluid prevents complete laser penetration to adequately treat the occult CNV component of the PED. While the 689-nm wavelength emitted by the laser activating verteporfin may not theoretically penetrate the serous fluid, the hypoperfusion spot following treatment is strong evidence against this theory.

Figure 10-5. An 81-year-old male with an occult CNV complaining of decreased visual acuity measured at 20/50. Stippled hyperfluorescence is evident on fluorescein angiography (A), and a

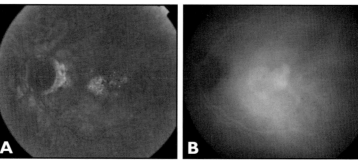

hyperfluorescent plaque is present on indocyanine green (B). A shallow PED is present on OCT (C) with intra- and subretinal fluid. The OCT map (D) demonstrates the area of subretinal fluid within the macula.

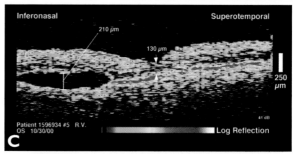

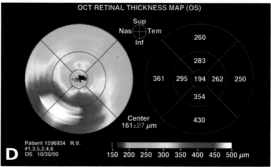

Maintenance of visual acuity is a factor of the integrity of the overlying RPE and retina. The OCT in serous PEDs demonstrates a relatively undisturbed RPE layer with no evidence of intraretinal fluid in this example. Our experience with other cases of serous PEDs is similar to this case, with immediate reduction in the serous cavity of the PED followed by reaccumulation of fluid. While the visual acuity typically improves, the clinical and angiographic picture remains relatively unchanged. More patients must be treated with longer follow-up to accurately conclude whether PDT effectively treats serous PEDs or if the lesions are following the natural history of disease.

OCCULT CHOROIDAL NEOVASCULARIZATION

An 81-year-old male with a disciform scar OD and chronic, stable occult CNV OS complained of dimming vision in his left eye. Examination revealed a shallow, fibrovascular PED with associated subretinal fluid. Visual acuity declined from 20/40 2 months prior to presentation to 20/50 on current examination. Fluorescein angiography demonstrated stippled hyperfluorescence with a hyperfluorescent plaque on indocyanine green angiography con-

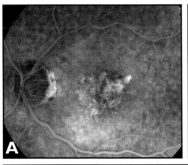

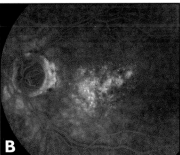

Figure 10-6. Nearly 3 months after treatment, the visual acuity was stable at 20/60. Stippled hyperfluorescence remained unchanged on fluorescein angiography in mid (A) and late frames (B). The OCT shows resolution of the intraretinal fluid with minimal residual subretinal fluid (C, D).

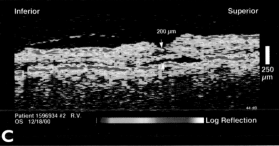

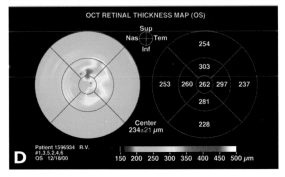

sistent with occult CNV. A shallow PED with intra- and subretinal fluid was visible on OCT (Figure 10-5). Given his functional monocular status with a disciform scar in the right eye, the patient elected to proceed with PDT. One month following treatment, the visual acuity measured 20/60 and the fluorescein angiography remained stable with stippled hyperfluorescence. Three months after treatment, the patient noted a subjective improvement while the vision remained stable at 20/60. The fluorescein angiography was unchanged and the OCT demonstrated a reduction of subretinal fluid with resolution of intraretinal fluid (Figure 10-6).

While PDT induces involution of CNV, persistence of the fibrotic component of the CNV remaining anterior to the RPE cell layer appears to limit visual recovery following treatment in classic lesions. The fibrotic lesion is visible clinically and angiographically and is represented by a highly reflective layer anterior to the RPE/choriocapillaris band on OCT. Compared to intraretinal CNV (Type II CNV), occult CNV remains underneath the RPE cell layer (Type I CNV). Therefore, any fibrosis remaining after treatment lies underneath the retina, providing an unobstructed pathway for light to reach the photoreceptors.

The Treatment of Age-Related Macular Degeneration with Photodynamic Therapy

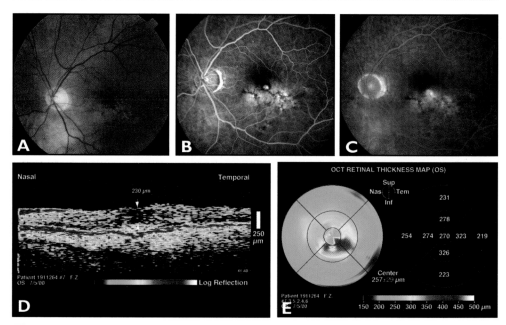

Figure 10-7. Color photograph (A) and fluorescein angiography (B) in a female with pattern dystrophy and visual acuity measuring 20/400. There is a focus of early hyperfluorescence surrounded by a hypofluorescent rim. Venous phase of the angiogram demonstrates leakage of fluorescein (C). Intraretinal fluid with loss of a normal foveal contour is present on OCT (D, E). The patient was treated with PDT.

(TAP) Study Group inadvertently treated a small subset of eyes with complete occult CNV. Of this subset, 36% of the verteporfin-treated eyes experienced moderate visual loss compared to 69% of placebo-treated eyes. Despite the difference, the number of patients enrolled was too small to reach a statistically significant result.[1]

The Verteporfin in Photodynamic Therapy (VIP) Study Group further evaluated the treatment of occult CNV with PDT in a randomized, multicenter, blinded clinical trial comparing verteporfin to placebo.[10] Qualifying occult lesions were less than 5400 microns in greatest linear dimension (GLD) extending under the foveal avascular zone, visual acuity of 20/100 or better. Hemorrhage associated with the lesion or documented deterioration in visual acuity (loss of at least 1 line) within the preceding 3 months. Deterioration was defined as loss of 1 line of visual acuity (five letters) or a 10% increase in the GLD of the lesion. Verteporfin was administered by standard TAP protocol.

While the VIP Study Group failed to demonstrate a benefit of verteporfin for the treatment of occult CNV at 12 months, a statistically significant benefit was identified at 24 months when compared to the natural history of disease.[10] Subgroup analysis of the occult group with no classic component discovered that the treatment benefit was greater for patients with either smaller lesions (≤ four disc areas) or visual acuity of 20/50 or worse. A 4% risk of severe visual loss within 7 days of treatment was noted only in the verteporfin-treated group. Clinical findings associated with this visual loss included the formation of subretinal pigment epithelial blood and marked subretinal fluid with choroidal hypofluorescence.[10] Complete results of the VIP Report #2 is discussed in detail in Chapter Six.

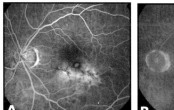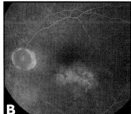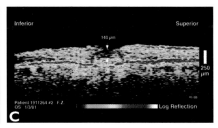

Figure 10-8. Fluorescein angiography 6 months following PDT demonstrates staining of fibrotic CNV surrounded by a rim of hypofluorescence (a) without late leakage (b). Restoration of a normal retinal contour is present with minimal subretinal fibrosis on OCT (c). Visual acuity improved to 20/40.

Lesion selection may have affected the visual outcome, preventing an earlier statistically significant result in the VIP Study Group. Qualifying lesions had to demonstrate either enlargement of the lesion or hemorrhage prior to enrollment. The presence of hemorrhage and exudation tends to imply a more chronic lesion with underlying fibrosis in the authors' experience. The hemorrhage appears to occur secondary to contraction of the fibrotic component, leading to shearing of surrounding vessels. Other factors that block fluorescence, such as exudation, also represent a sign of chronicity. In our experience with classic lesions, treatment of CNV with a component of fibrosis responds poorly to PDT with verteporfin (see Chapter Nine). It may be that the VIP Study Group selected lesions that were too chronic to favorably respond sooner to PDT with verteporfin. When deciding to initiate treatment of occult lesions, the authors rely more on subjective visual loss, as this tends to identify an active lesion. Earlier treatment may subtend better anatomic and visual results. OCT is also a useful adjunct to treatment, as intraretinal and subretinal fluid tends to be present in active occult lesions, with resolution of the fluid following successful treatment.

As described in Chapter Four, diode laser photocoagulation of occult lesions is currently under investigation in the Transpupillary Thermotherapy for Occult Subfoveal Choroidal Neovascularization (TTT4CNV).

PATTERN DYSTROPHY

A 76-year-old female with pattern dystrophy presented with a 2-week history of metamorphopsia OS and visual acuity measuring 20/400. Fluorescein angiography identified a subfoveal CNV with accumulation of intraretinal fluid on OCT (Figure 10-7). PDT with verteporfin was performed with a 2000-micron spot. One month following treatment, the visual acuity improved to 20/50 with resolution of subretinal fluid on examination. Visual acuity stabilized at 20/40 6 months following treatment. Staining of subretinal fibrosis was present on fluorescein angiography (Figure 10-8), and the intraretinal fluid resolved with restoration of normal retinal contour on OCT.

INDOCYANINE GREEN HOT SPOTS

A 71-year-old male with AMD presented with 5 days of decreased visual acuity in the left eye measuring 20/400. Subretinal fluid, hemorrhage, and early fibrosis were present on funduscopic examination. Occult CNV was identified on fluorescein angiography with obscu-

Figure 10-9. A 79-year-old male presented with subfoveal CNV OS (A). Fluorescein angiography reveals leakage of fluorescein with obscuration of the entire lesion from scattered hemorrhage (B, C). There is a focal area of hyperfluorescence on indocyanine green angiography, referred to as an indocyanine green hot spot (D). Subretinal fluid is present on OCT (E, F). Visual acuity measured 20/400.

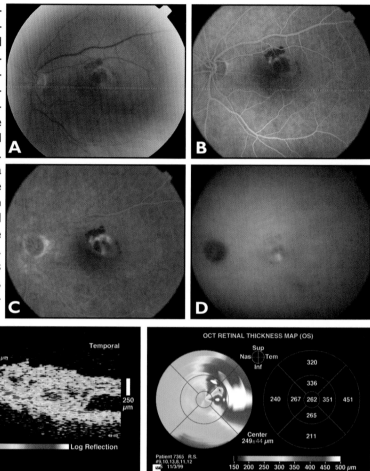

ration of the lesion borders by blood. A focal area of hyperfluorescence (indocyanine green hot spot) was identified on indocyanine green angiography (Figure 10-9). PDT using verteporfin was performed with a spot size encompassing the entire lesion, including the indocyanine green hot spot. Twelve days following PDT, the vision improved to 20/60 with diminished subretinal fluid and restoration of a near normal foveal contour on OCT. The CNV was hypoperfused on fluorescein angiography with elimination of the focal hot spot on indocyanine green angiography (Figure 10-10). Angiography performed 3 and 6 months following treatment demonstrated resolution of the hemorrhage with persistence of stippled hyperfluorescence consistent with occult CNV. The indocyanine green hot spot remained absent. Fourteen months following initial treatment, the visual acuity remained 20/60 with stable fluorescein and indocyanine green angiography (Figure 10-11).

Indocyanine green angiography is a useful tool in delineating occult CNV. In 1000 consecutive eyes with occult CNV identified on fluorescein angiography, Guyer et al[11] further classified these lesions using indocyanine green. Three distinct morphologic types of occult CNV were identified on indocyanine green angiography, which included plaques, focal spots, and lesions with a combination of both plaques and spots. Focal spots (indocyanine

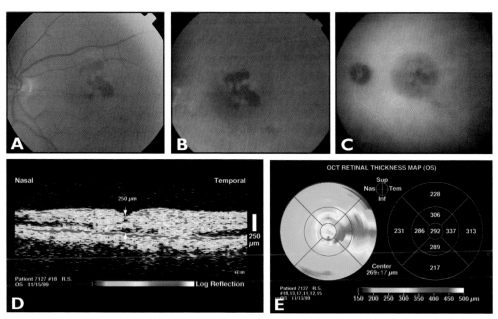

Figure 10-10. Two weeks following PDT with verteporfin, the visual acuity improved to 20/60 (A). A hypofluorescent treatment spot is identified on both fluorescein (B) and indocyanine green angiography (C). There has been a slight expansion of the subretinal hemorrhage, but the CNV is nonperfused and the indocyanine green hot spot is absent. There is restoration of a normal fovea contour on cross-sectional OCT (D) with resolution of the subretinal fluid on the OCT map (E).

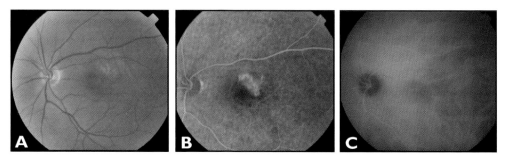

Figure 10-11. Six months following PDT, the visual acuity was 20/60 (A). On fluorescein angiography, stippled hyperfluorescence consistent with an occult CNV is visible (B), as the subretinal hemorrhage visible in Figures 10-9 and 10-10 have cleared (A). The indocyanine green angiography was hypofluorescent in the area of the previous indocyanine green hot spot (C).

green hot spots) are areas of bright fluorescence of less than 1 disc area. Plaques are defined as areas of hyperfluorescence on indocyanine green angiography that are greater than 1 disc area and usually subfoveal. Plaques may be well defined with discrete borders or poorly defined with irregular borders. The hyperfluorescence is typically less intense than that observed with focal spots. Plaques were identified in 61% and focal spots in 29% of the eyes

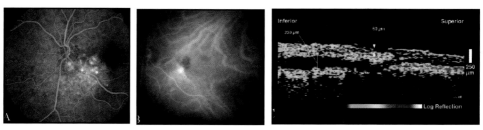

Figure 10-12. Visual acuity measured counting fingers in this 74-year-old female with PCV. Fluorescein angiography demonstrates the polypoidal areas of hyperfluorescence with leakage and a focal area of intense hyperfluorescence on indocyanine green. The OCT demonstrates subretinal fluid with the reflective signal in the fovea representing exudation.

imaged. Combination lesions with a focal spot adjacent, overlying, or remote from the plaque were observed in only 8% of eyes with occult CNV.

The natural history of focal indocyanine green spots is unknown.[4,5] As indocyanine green hot spots are usually extrafoveal, Slakter and associates evaluated 79 eyes with focal spots treated by indocyanine green-guided laser photocoagulation.[12] With a median follow-up of 23 weeks, 56% of eyes had complete resolution of exudative findings, 15% had partial resolution, and 29% of the 79 eyes experienced persistence or worsening of exudative manifestations. Forty-three percent had one or more episodes of recurrence during the study. The median visual acuity measured 20/200. Thirteen percent of eyes improved by more than 2 lines of Snellen visual acuity with stabilization in 53%. When comparing eyes with or without a serous PED, eyes without a serous PED demonstrated a slightly more favorable result with respect to anatomic outcome, recurrence rate, and visual improvement than those with a serous PED.

The use of PDT in the above example effectively treated the indocyanine green hot spot. However, the entire occult CNV was treated in addition to the focal spot. The large spot size may have attributed to the success in this case. Longer follow-up and more cases are required to adequately evaluate the efficacy of PDT of indocyanine green hot spots.

POLYPOIDAL CHOROIDAL VASCULOPATHY

A 74-year-old white female presented with decreased visual acuity to counting fingers in her left eye for approximately 2 weeks. On funduscopic examination OD there was a small, punctate, orange-red lesion along the inferior temporal arcade without hemorrhage or exudation. Examination OS revealed exudation originating from the peripapillary area around the inferior temporal arcade with associated subretinal fluid. Multiple focal areas of hyperfluorescence were visible on fluorescein angiography with an intense focal area of hyperfluorescence on indocyanine green. OCT corroborated the clinical findings of subretinal fluid and demonstrated the foveal exudation (Figure 10-12). A diagnosis of PCV was made. Given the poor visual prognosis from exudation involving the fovea and the choroidal vascular nature of the disease, PDT with verteporfin was performed with a 5000-micron spot centered on the inferior temporal arcade, extending to the edge of foveal exudation, and avoiding the optic nerve. A subjective improvement in visual acuity was noted 2 weeks following treatment with acuity measured at 20/40 at 1 month. Three months after treatment, the acuity improved to 20/30 with clinical resolution of the subretinal fluid. The polypoidal

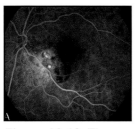
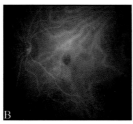
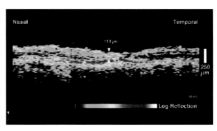

Figure 10-13. Three months following PDT with verteporfin, the visual acuity improved to 20/30. The polypoidal lesions are fewer in number and stain on fluorescein angiography without late leakage. The indocyanine green angiography demonstrates a hypofluorescent spot secondary to persistent exudation, with disappearance of the hyperfluorescent area of leakage present prior to treatment. On OCT there is resolution of the subretinal fluid with persistent hard exudate represented by the highly reflective red band in the fovea.

lesions appeared inactive on fluorescein angiography with staining and absence of leakage, and the indocyanine green angiography demonstrated resolution of the hyperfluorescent lesion in the macula. OCT mirrored the clinical exam with resolution of the subretinal fluid and persistent exudation (Figure 10-13). The visual acuity remains stable without requiring retreatment on further examinations.

PCV is an abnormality of the choroidal vasculature characterized by dilated choroidal vessels terminating in aneurysmal swelling in a polypoidal configuration. The abnormal vasculature is typically bilateral and located in the peripapillary region, but abnormal vessels may be identified in the macula. Clinically, orange-red punctate lesions representing polypoidal vessels are visible on biomicroscopy. However, these visible polypoidal lesions are usually masked by large serous and hemorrhagic detachments of the RPE and neurosensory retina. The average visual acuity has been reported to be about 20/80, and the patients have a better prognosis than those with AMD. The imaging study of choice is indocyanine green angiography, which demonstrates the abnormal vessels in the early phase of the study. Fluorescein angiography is also useful for delineating the abnormal vasculature, as is seen in the previous case report.[13,14]

Unless hemorrhage or exudation threatens the macula with decreased visual acuity, most patients are conservatively managed with observation. Argon laser photocoagulation is the most common mode of treatment with laser applied to the extrafoveal abnormal vasculature. Diode laser photocoagulation has also been described in one case report.[14] Shiraga and associates[16] treated eight eyes with thick submacular hemorrhage using pars plana vitrectomy and tissue plasminogen activator-assisted removal of subretinal blood. Laser was then applied to the extrafoveal abnormal vasculature in four eyes. Visual acuity improved or stabilized in seven of eight eyes, with one eye experiencing a decline in visual acuity secondary to the formation of CNV.

Angioid Streaks

A 52-year-old female presented with a sudden onset of visual loss in her left eye. Visual acuity measured 20/200, and a diagnosis of angioid streaks with associated CNV was made. Angiography demonstrated a classic CNV with a greatest linear dimension of 4400 mm (Figure 10-14 [A]). Significant intra- and subretinal fluid was identified on OCT.

Figure 10-14. A 52-year-old female with angioid streaks presented with CNV in her left eye associated with surrounding subretinal hemorrhage. Visual acuity measured 20/200 and PDT with verteporfin was performed (A). One month following PDT angiography demonstrates decreased hemorrhage with minimal leakage from the treated CNV (B). She returned 5 months following initial PDT with visual acuity of 20/400 and increased leakage from recurrent CNV (C). The lesion was retreated and the patient was lost to follow-up for 7 months. Fluorescein angiography 1 year from the initial treatment and 7 months after retreatment shows staining of the CNV with no active leakage (D). Visual acuity improved to 20/125 and no further treatment was performed. Cystoid macular edema was present on OCT (not shown).

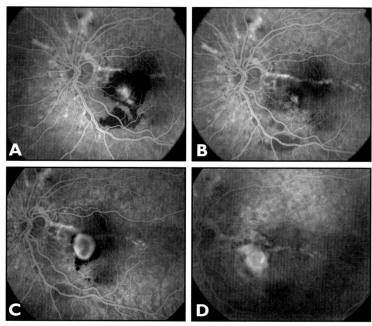

Photodynamic therapy was performed with subsequent improvement in visual acuity and reduction in intraretinal fluid 1 month following treatment. Angiography did demonstrate a small area of hyperfluorescence but given the dramatic reduction in macular thickness, the lesion was observed (Figure 10-14 [B]). Five months after the initial treatment, visual acuity declined to 20/400 with recurrence of the CNV on fluorescein angiography (Figure 10-14 [C]). Repeat PDT was performed with a 3500 mm spot size. The patient was lost to follow-up for 7 months and returned noting a recent improvement in her visual acuity, measuring 20/125. The prior CNV was inactive and closed on fluorescein angiography with vision reduced from cystoid macular edema identified on OCT (Figure 10-14 [D]). No further intervention was offered and the patient continues to be observed.

The authors have collectively treated five eyes of five patients with verteporfin for CNV from angioid streaks. The mean age was 61.5 years (range: 52 to 78) with a mean follow-up of 8 months (range: 5 to 11 months). The initial lesion was subfoveal in four eyes and juxtafoveal in one eye. Only one eye demonstrated an improvement in visual acuity (patient described above). The mean pretreatment visual acuity was 20/250, with a mean post-treatment visual acuity of 20/325. Three eyes required two treatments with one eye receiving a total of three treatments.[17]

More conventional treatments have showed only limited promise as well. Laser photocoagulation may be used for juxtafoveal and extrafoveal lesions, but no benefit has been established for laser photocoagulation of subfoveal lesions.[18,19] Results of submacular surgery have also been disappointing.[20] A preliminary study of PDT using verteporfin for treatment of CNV secondary to causes other than AMD treated one eye with angioid streaks.[21] The visual acuity remained stable at its pretreatment level of 20/64. However, the duration of follow-up was only 12 weeks. While the five patients in our series who were treated with PDT are limited in number and duration of follow-up, the visual results are not encouraging. A larger series of patients is necessary to draw any conclusions on whether PDT is effective for the treatment of CNV from angioid streaks.

IDIOPATHIC CNV

The authors have treated six patients with idiopathic CNV. All were woman under 60 years of age. Of all the patients treated with PDT using verteporfin, this subgroup of younger women responded the most favorably to treatment. Patients were typically treated with a 1-week course of oral steroids without clinical improvement followed immediately by PDT. Visual acuity either stabilized or improved in all treated eyes. One retreatment was typically required before stabilization of the CNV. This represents one of our most successfully treated subgroups of eyes. While these results are encouraging, they may not represent any alteration in the natural history of the disease, as described in Chapter Two.

CONCLUSION

While the TAP and VIP Studies have identified specific subgroups of patients that benefit from PDT, its application is currently limited. Clearly, the use of PDT to treat vascular disorders will be expanded in the future. Further case reports and randomized trials will be necessary to identify which disorders benefit from photodynamic therapy.

REFERENCES

1. Treatment of Age-Related Macular Degeneration with Photodynamic Therapy (TAP) Study Group. Photodynamic therapy of subfoveal choroidal neovascularization in age-related macular degeneration with verteporfin. *Arch Ophthalmol.* 1999;117:1329-1345.

2. Treatment of Age-Related Macular Degeneration with Photodynamic Therapy (TAP) Study Group. Photodynamic therapy of subfoveal choroidal neovascularization in age-related macular degeneration with verteporfin: two-year results of two randomized clinical trials—TAP report #2. In press.

3. Poliner LS, Olk RJ, Burgess D, et al. Natural history of pigment epithelial detachment in age-related macular degeneration. *Ophthalmology.* 1986;93:543-551.

4. Meredith TA, Braley RE, Aaberg TM. Natural history of serous pigment epithelial detachments of the retinal pigment epithelium. *Am J Ophthalmol.* 1979;88:643-651.

5. Casswell AG, Kohen D, Bird AC. Retinal pigment epithelial detachments in the elderly: classification and outcome. *Br J Ophthalmol.* 1985;69:397-403.

6. Bird AC. Recent advances in the treatment of senile disciform macular degeneration by photocoagulation. *Br J Ophthalmol.* 1974;58:367-376.

7. Braunstein RA, Gass JDM. Serous detachments of the retinal pigment epithelium in patients with senile macular disease. *Am J Ophthalmol.* 1979;88:652-660.

8. The Moorfields Macular Study Group. Retinal pigment epithelial detachments in the elderly: a controlled trial of argon laser photocoagulation. *Br J Ophthalmol.* 1982;66:1-16.

9. Barondes MJ, Pagliarini S, Chisholm IH, et al. Controlled trial of laser photocoagulation of pigment epithelial detachments in the elderly: 4 year review. *Br J Ophthalmol.* 1992;75:5-7.

10. Verteporfin in Photodynamic Therapy (VIP) Study Group. Verteporfin therapy of subfoveal choroidal

neovascularization in age-related macular degeneration: two-year results of a randomized clinical trial including lesions with occult but no classic neovascularization—VIP report #2. *Am J Ophthalmol.* 2001;131:541-560.

11. Guyer DR, Yannuzzi LA, Slakter JS, et al. Classification of choroidal neovascularization by digital indocyanine green videoangiography. *Ophthalmology.* 1996;103:2054-2060.

12. Slakter JS, Yannuzzi LA, Sorenson JA, et al. A pilot study of indocyanine green videoangiography-guided laser photocoagulation of occult choroidal neovascularization in age-related macular degeneration. *Arch Ophthalmol.* 1994;112:465-472.

13. Yannuzzi LA, Ciardella A, Spaide RF, et al. The expanding clinical spectrum of idiopathic polypoidal choroidal vasculopathy. *Arch Ophthalmol.* 1997;115:478-485.

14. Yannuzzi LA, Wong DWK, Sforzolini BS, et al. Polypoidal choroidal vasculopathy and neovascularized age-related macular degeneration. *Arch Ophthalmol.* 1999;117:1503-1510.

15. Gomez-Ulla F, Gonzalez F, Torreiro MG. Diode laser photocoagulation in idiopathic polypoidal choroidal vasculopathy. *Retina.* 1998;18:481-483.

16. Shiraga F, Matsuo T, Yokoe S, et al. Surgical treatment of submacular hemorrhage associated with idiopathic polypoidal choroidal vasculopathy. *Am J Ophthalmol.* 1999;128:147-154.

17. Greenberg PB, Rogers A, Martidis A, et al. Photodynamic therapy with verteporfin for choroidal neovascularization due to angioid streaks. *Invest Ophthalmol Vis Sci.* 2001;42:S440.

18. Gelisken O, Hendrikse F, Deutman AF. A long-term follow-up study of laser coagulation of neovascular membranes in angioid streaks. *Am J Ophthalmol.* 1988;105:299-303.

19. Lim JI, Bressler NM, Marsh MJ, Bressler SB. Laser treatment of choroidal neovascularization in patients with angioid streaks. *Am J Ophthalmol.* 1993;116:414-423.

20. Adelberg DA, Del Priore LV, Kaplan HJ. Surgery for subfoveal membranes in myopia, angioid streaks and other disorders. *Retina.* 1995;15:198-205.

21. Sickenberg M, Schmidt-Erfurth U, Miller JW, et al. A preliminary study of photodynamic therapy using verteporfin for choroidal neovascularization in pathologic myopia, ocular histoplasmosis syndrome, angioid streaks, and idiopathic causes. *Arch Ophthalmol.* 2000;117:327-36.

INDEX

BUILD *Your Library*

This book and many others on numerous different topics are available from SLACK Incorporated. For further information or a copy of our latest catalog, contact us at:

Professional Book Division
SLACK Incorporated
6900 Grove Road
Thorofare, NJ 08086 USA
Telephone: 1-856-848-1000
1-800-257-8290
Fax: 1-856-853-5991
E-mail: orders@slackinc.com
www.slackbooks.com

We accept most major credit cards and checks or money orders in US dollars drawn on a US bank. Most orders are shipped within 72 hours.

Contact us for information on recent releases, forthcoming titles, and bestsellers. If you have a comment about this title or see a need for a new book, direct your correspondence to the Editorial Director at the above address.

Thank you for your interest and we hope you found this work beneficial.